What others say...

"This book is a great resource for parents who are being introduced into the world of children with behavioral problems. For parents this situation can be terrifying.

Many parents initially respond with fear when they learn their child has issues they do not understand. The child typically responds with anger, even if that reaction is not always visible. Since anger is a secondary emotion to an underlying problem, the ability to identify the source of the anger becomes very important for parents. As Dr. Davick talks about in Chapter One, recognizing miskidding and learning to manage it effectively can determine the difference in the path a child takes to adulthood.

This book identifies critical methods toward managing some problematic behavior. It makes clear the importance of understanding and either seeking effective and helpful treatment to change the behavior or accepting the behavior and learning to live with it.

In my professional and personal opinion making one of these two choices will create a sense of choice and control for the child in a situation where there are no real choices.

Dr. Davick does an excellent job in his book helping parents to learn to understand the importance of recognizing and dealing with these children's issues without increasing their fear and anger. This book also helps parents identify dangerous behavior that cannot be ignored, which he calls KILLER KIDDING, without causing a panic response which can alienate a child and lead to further problems.

Dr.Davick breaks down complex theories and behavior dynamics into easy-to-understand charts and tables.

Overall this book was a pleasure to read with an organized flow. He creates simplicity for issues that in most situations appear to be an insurmountable obstacle."

~Laura Youngfleisch, Masters of Arts (MA), Licensed Mental Health Counselor (LMHC)

"Dr. Davick, drawing on over 40 years' experience, has produced a tool that helps parents recognize, analyze, and modify unwanted behaviors from the cradle to the day an adolescent leaves home. With thoughtfulness and expertise, he has devised a method to distinguish healthy exploration and experimentation from behaviors that lead to unwanted consequences. And, with many practical illustrations, he suggests the most useful behavior modification methods that emphasize the consequences of children's actions when necessary (as well as assessing when intervention is unnecessary). Miskidding is not a reference book to gather dust on the shelf; it's a readable book that everyone supervising children will enjoy for its useful tips and easy to understand system: an extraordinary addition to the arsenal of tools available for all who care for and about kids."

~Bennett E. Werner, M.D.

Fellow of the American College of Physicians

"My first reaction is 'wow, he has obviously put a lot of work into this!' It's a very ambitious project - you are trying to create new nomenclature and frameworks, and the act of defining and explaining them is very difficult (but ultimately could be how this work actually changes the dialog for the better in this area)."

~Christopher Baugh, M.D., M.B.A., Brigham & Women's Hospital, Boston, MA

Managing *Mis*behavior in Kids:
The *Mis*Kidding® Process

Alan M. Davick, M.D.

Managing *Mis*behavior in Kids: The *Mis*Kidding® Process
Alan M. Davick, M.D.

© 2013 Alan M. Davick, M.D.

ISBN: 978-0-9890053-0-2

MISKIDDING, LLC
P.O. Box 101127
Cape Coral, FL 33910-1127

URL: www.miskidding.com
Email: miskidding1@gmail.com

Disclaimer:

This book is intended to be a guide to recognizing and managing misbehavior in children. It is not intended to be a recipe for diagnosing or treating physical or mental illness, nor does the purchase of this book establish in any way a professional relationship with the author or publisher.

The author and publisher are not responsible for the use or non-use of any diagnostic procedure, treatment option or choice of medication mentioned in this book. The reader is cautioned that new information regarding diagnostic procedures, treatment options and medication-related information accumulates daily and may render the examples presented in this book outdated or even contraindicated by the date of publication. Therefore, the author and publisher do not assume and hereby disclaim any liability to any party for any loss, damage or disruption caused by error or omission in this book and associated websites or videos.

This book and associated websites and videos are not intended to replace medical, neurological, genetic, psychological or psychiatric advice tendered by the reader's own professional consultant(s) and the reader is strongly advised to discuss any pending decisions regarding diagnosis, treatment options or medication with such consultants.

Cover graphics:
© Dmytro Rozumeyenko | Dreamstime.com
© Alexandre Zveiger | Dreamstime.com
© Jose Manuel Gelpi Diaz | Dreamstime.com
© Anke Van Wyk | Dreamstime.com

Cover design:
Rik Feeney / Rik@PublishingSuccessOnline.com

ACKNOWLEDGMENTS

The *MIS/kidding*® **Process** was developed over many years by a painstaking collection of *pearls of wisdom and expertise* from colleagues in the fields of Medicine, Psychology and Education as well as from interaction with a myriad of families. A complete listing of all those who influenced this effort would require several books of this size! Nevertheless, the author shall attempt to list some of those peers with whom he had the honor and pleasure of working and who, by their example, contributed to the writing of this book.

Physicians

Dr. Don Baracski, Adolescent & Adult Psychiatrist, Chief Medical Officer, Lee Mental Health

Dr. Arnold Capute, Behavioral-Developmental Pediatrician

Dr. George Dover, Pediatrician-in-Chief, Johns Hopkins Medical Institutions

Dr. Victor Ferrans, Adolescent & Adult Psychiatrist

Dr. James Harrison, Child & Adolescent Psychiatrist

Dr. Dan Levy, Behavioral-Developmental Pediatrician

Dr. Lawrence C. Pakula, Behavioral-Developmental Pediatrician

Dr. Alejandro Rodriguez, Child Psychiatrist

Psychologists & Social Workers

Dr. George Dorry, Psychologist

Dr. Anna Rosenberg, Psychologist

Dr. Leon Rosenberg, Psychologist

Dr. Sandra Rosenblatt, Psychologist

Stuart Tiegel, Social Worker

Laura Youngfleisch, Social Worker

Educators

Dr. Susan Grant, Neurolinguist

Dr. Nancy Grasmick, Former MD Superintendent of Schools

The author would like to recognize the critical contributions of Rik Feeney, author, publisher, editor and coach, under whose direction and unfailing professionalism this book took shape. Fortunately, Rik's many talents include an expert knowledge of gymnastics, enabling him to contort to the demands of this unruly manuscript.

Finally, my everlasting love and gratitude to Barbara, my window on the "real" world.

Al Davick

Dedication

Managing Misbehavior in Kids: The *Mis*/Kidding® Process

This book is dedicated to my creators:

- My Heavenly Father, who breathed life into me and gifted me with a bit of insight
- Dr. Irvin and Sylvia Davick, who instilled in me a love of learning and a sensitivity to the suffering of others
- Dr. Alejandro Rodriguez, who taught me to observe like a Pediatrician and to think like a Psychiatrist

Table of Contents

PREFACE

Late in 1972, I had completed training as a Pediatrician at Johns Hopkins and was supplementing that experience with an additional year of Fellowship in Child Psychiatry. One day, I was called to the office of Dr. Alejandro Rodriguez, my mentor and Chief of the Department of Child Psychiatry. Alejandro had a project in mind. He wanted someone to write a manual for child-oriented professionals. The idea was to help organize the thinking of behavioral consultants, the professionals who face terrified parents, frustrated teachers or bewildered counselors. The book would guide those professionals through the steps of deciding if a child's behavior was normal or abnormal, if it had to be controlled then and there or over a period of time, if it had a physical basis or not and how to alleviate the problem. Alejandro wanted me to write that manual.

There was certainly a need for the book. As a novice Pediatrician I had already struggled with behaviors in children that were difficult to assign to the "organic" (physical) or the "functional" (mental) categories. As a Child Psychiatric Fellow I was consulted frequently to make such determinations. Even at that stage in my development I could see the outlines of a "process" that would lead to the diagnosis and management of these behaviors. Part of the process involved history taking, a skill upon which Pediatricians lavish much attention. Though physical and neurological examinations were usually performed on each child, along with occasional laboratory tests, these rarely contributed much to an understanding of problem behaviors. Having taken detailed histories, performed meticulous physical examinations and ordered sophisticated laboratory tests, pediatric residents usually sought guidance from one of the "masters", like Alejandro or one of his peers. These experienced clinicians included Psychologists and Psychiatric Social Workers as well as Psychiatrists. We could observe them as they observed and ministered to children and parents. Some of them were consistently effective, others not so. It was up to us as trainees to discern their methodology, but the wide variety of techniques employed and the fact that some of the most effective clinicians were among the least gifted teachers left us in the dark when we tried to reconstruct their techniques.

As medical students have done for centuries, we ascribed this advanced clinical acumen to "intuition", a "sixth sense" acquired only after years of clinical practice. We residents and fellows relied upon our physical and laboratory machinations to fill in gaps in our own "intuitive" skills, though they rarely did. To write a book about such an ethereal process seemed impossible, certainly at that stage in my professional development. I declined Alejandro's suggestion and completed my studies.

More than forty years have passed since those days in training. As a Behavioral Pediatrician, I've consulted daily with parents and their professional helpers as they've tried to distinguish aberrant behaviors due to physical disease, including psychosis, from manipulative behaviors due to children's' inappropriate choice-making. These many years of practice at the interface between parents, teachers and professionals have taught me much about the process used by my former preceptors. I have learned to teach the process to parents and to fellow professionals. Most important, I've discovered that parents can successfully manage their children's' behaviors without delegating their authority to professionals. To do so, they must be empowered by knowledge of practical criteria for recognizing *mis*/behaviors and by access (though not submission) to professional assistance.

In daily practice, during a typical brief behavioral consultation with a parent, it isn't possible or desirable to transform the consultee into a Behavioral Pediatrician. The first order of business is to put the parent at ease; to assuage guilt, to change a frame of mind from terror and impotence to one of opportunity within a professional partnership. To accomplish this, three obstacles must be removed from a parent's path. These behavioral fallacies, taken to extremes, become idiocies which enable the growth of misbehavior. I call them the Permissive Idiocy, the Protective Idiocy and the Professional Idiocy. A bit of exaggeration will acquaint you with them and show you their absurdity:

Permissive Idiocy:

1. Behavior has no discernible cause. It's *mysterious*, spontaneous, magical and uncontrollable. Behavior is the expression of children's' inalienable right to do as they please.

2. *Children know better than adults* whether their behavior is acceptable.

3. The world (including teachers and the community at large) MUST ADJUST to children's' behaviors because their parents have.

4. Controlling misbehavior *breaks the spirit* and leads to a *squashed*, perhaps even to an *obliterated* mind. By contrast, allowing outrageous misbehavior permits the growth of "natural inclinations", a free mind, and *spunk*.

Protective Idiocy:

1. Children are too *frail* and too *dumb* to learn from the consequences of their behaviors.

2. Children who are allowed to suffer the consequences of their own acts *think their parents don't love them.*

3. Parents and other adults must show their love by protecting children from the consequences of their misbehaviors.

The Permissive Idiocy assumes that parents can't figure out what children are doing and why, and that controlling their behaviors will somehow seriously hurt them. The Protective Idiocy assumes children can't or won't figure out why adults make them follow rules and that the result will be their loss of love for parents. These assumptions are so threatening that they lead to an over reliance on professionals for managing children's' behaviors, the last of the idiocies.

Professional Idiocy:

1. *Only Professionals* can recognize and solve behavior problems in children without hurting them or turning off their love.

2. Professionals know the *truth* about behavior and love (indeed, the truth about everything).

3. Professionals (who know the truth) *cannot be fired*, nor can their competence or success in solving problems be measured.

The Professional Idiocy confuses knowledge with wisdom. True, professionals have studied forever, hold degrees and have gained much knowledge about why children behave as they do, but those who believe this idiocy assume that only people with such knowledge can decide what is a problem and why. Ignored is the fact that professionals and children are often least steeped in wisdom. The first group, because they've been in school so long, have had too few life experiences to guide them, while the second group are too young to have acquired them!

After the idiocies have been demolished as obstacles to a parent's control, a basic understanding of the worrisome behavior and a safe, timely and effective strategy for controlling it must be developed. This, I have learned, is best accomplished by demystifying the process of behavioral management.

In this book, I've established a hierarchy of reverence. Though I revere children and respect their goals, I revere adults and their goals for children even more, certainly for most of childhood. Hence, in *MIS*/KIDDING, as a reminder of this hierarchy, I irreverently refer to children as kids. To demystify kids' behaviors, I refer to everything kids do as kidding and all their misbehaviors as *mis*/kidding.

MIS/KIDDING® is written in six chapters. The first five chapters show you an easy five-step process you can use to recognize and control any degree of *mis*/kidding. The steps of this process are presented in sequence as three diagnostic chapters and two management chapters. A sixth chapter "puts it all together" and gives you some experience applying these steps to *mis*/kidding problems.

In reading this book, imagine you've come to my office to talk with me about your kids. We've met each other here in the Preface. Now come with me through the Introduction and find a comfortable chair. Then, sit back and let me teach you what you need to know about *mis*/kidding.

Alan M. Davick, M.D.
Cape Coral, FL

INTRODUCTION

Kidding is all the things kids can be seen to do or not do. Good/kidding is acceptable or normal kidding and *mis*/kidding is unacceptable or abnormal kidding. No matter whether kids are moving or still, noisy or silent, awake or asleep, they're always "kidding."

There's always a reason for kidding. From scientists who see how changes in brain chemistry make an arm move, to teachers who see Johnny pull Sally's hair and get poked in return, we live day to day knowing the things kids do have reasons behind them. Though the scientists don't know why brain chemicals were released at that moment, they do know those chemicals allowed the brain to work and to move the muscles. Likewise, teachers don't know why Johnny pulled Sally's hair at that moment, but they do know that Sally poked Johnny in retaliation. We spend much of our time each day "reading" and reacting to kidding as if we understood the reasons behind it. We're all part-time behaviorists.

Sometimes, events cause what seems to be meaningless kidding that we can't read. Medical conditions like Epilepsy and Schizophrenia take away kids' choices for kidding. So do psychological and educational handicaps like Autism and Dyslexia. Whenever kidding seems meaningless, we can be sure there are hidden causes.

When handicapping conditions don't take away kids' choices, we can affect kidding by changing the reasons why kids chose the kidding. We can, in other words, make kids offers they can't refuse and thus give them better reasons for good/kidding than for *mis*/kidding.

This is a book about consequences. It's about recognizing the consequences of *mis*/kidding for kids and those around them. It's about devising consequences to influence or control kidding. Though the goals of kids and adults are often complementary, they're rarely identical. Kids need to find out who they are and how to conduct their lives. They do this by testing those around them. Adults want kids to grow up and become responsible. Kids need to know if this is worth doing. They scrutinize the consequences of their encounters with authority. At critical points, when the consequences of more mature behavior are compelling enough, kids move closer to adulthood by becoming more responsible.

You might ask, why the focus on *mis*/kidding rather than on good/kidding.

One reason for focusing on *mis*/kidding is that it often masks underlying limitations, either innate or those imposed by disease or other handicapping conditions. While parents need not worry if good/kidding springs from high motivation and hard work or is merely a manifestation of hidden talents, the management of *mis*/kidding is critically dependent on the recognition of hidden limitations and handicaps. Simple techniques for recognizing hidden causes are an integral part of *MIS*/KIDDING®.

Another reason for focusing on *mis*/kidding is because it's not until kids' behaviors create problems that parents and other authority persons reach for help. Good/kidding slowly moves kids toward adulthood. *Mis*/kidding moves kids away from adulthood and can even kill them. But the power of *mis*/kidding, when harnessed, can launch kids enormous distances toward maturity in a short time. After all, *mis*/kidding is really misdirected motivation. Helping kids use their own energies to achieve worthwhile goals is the epitome of parenting. That's why, in working with parents, I encourage them to view even the most severe *mis*/kidding episodes as fortuitous opportunities that can strengthen love and responsibility.

MIS/KIDDING® should not provoke you to try to control all kids' behaviors. It's impossible! Kids spend one hundred percent of their energies being kids. Parents can't (and shouldn't) attempt to devote that much energy to kid control. Besides, most of what kids do is simply kidding and requires no control. Your ultimate goal as a parent, and one which we'll work together to achieve through this book, is to get kids to control their own behaviors.

The next chapters present a few principles you need to know to identify and manage *mis*/kidding. Each of the next five chapters covers one of five steps you'll learn to use to recognize and control *mis*/kidding:

- Recognizing *mis*/kidding

- Determining the severity of the *mis*/kidding

- Deciding if you need professional help

- Substituting good/kidding goals

- Energizing the good/kidding

Along the way, we'll become acquainted with Physicians, Psychologists and Educators, three categories of professional helpers who recognize hidden conditions that kids can't control and assist you with difficult problems.

A sixth chapter presents a flow sheet to help you use this process to solve *mis*/kidding problems.

Some more technical information not of immediate use in applying the principles you learn in the first five chapters is presented in Part Three and the Appendices. For example, you review various physical conditions that cause *mis*/kidding and the different titles used by Physicians, Psychologists and Educators, the professionals who can and sometimes can't help your kid.

MIS/KIDDING® is meant to be read slowly, in a quiet room, no kids in sight or even within earshot. As you learn to use the powerful techniques that follow, you will take command of *mis*/kidding.

Now, find a tranquil spot. Put your feet up and read the Glossary where there are some terms you'll be learning about. Don't try to memorize them, just roll them on your tongue. Though they're all explained later, it's useful to see them all in one place for future reference.

GLOSSARY OF TERMS

KIDS: Children (who are not yet ready to accept full responsibility for the consequences of their acts).

KIDDING: Everything kids do. Behavior in kids.

- *Mis*/kidding:*Mis*behavior in kids. Undesirable kidding, defined by its ill consequences for kids or others.

- *KILLER*/kidding®: Severe *mis*/kidding, threatening injury or death to self or others, which must be STOPPED immediately.

- *Mid*/kidding:Moderately severe *mis*/kidding which leaves time for planning a strategy. Ignored, it becomes *KILLER*/kidding.

- mini/kidding: Mildly annoying *mis*/kidding, best ignored.

- Good/kidding: Constructive kidding that moves a kid along the path to adulthood. What kids do to achieve maturity and improve relationships to Others and those in Authority.

- In/kidding: Kidding created by processes within kids over which they have no control.

- Out/kidding: Kidding that kids choose to engage in.

- Active Out/kidding: Kids choosing to do things they're not supposed to do.

- Passive Out/kidding: Kids choosing not to do things they're supposed to do.

CONSEQUENCES:Events which occur spontaneously or which can be devised to influence Out/kidding.

- Reward: A pleasant consequence for kidding. It can promote good/kidding if given after it is earned. An especially powerful motivator when it takes the form of affection.

- Bribe: A "reward" given before it is earned. A dishonest and ineffective way to influence kidding.

- Punishment: A painful or unpleasant consequence. An efficient tool for stopping *mis*/kidding, it does not promote good/kidding because it makes kids angry or depressed.

CONSEQUENCE AREAS: The areas of life affected by kidding: Age Work, Others, Authority.

AGE WORK:Things kids must do at each stage of life to develop normally. A Consequence Area that includes physical, social and communication components. Failure to achieve any component of Age Work is an objective criterion of *mis*/kidding.

- physical skills:The part of Age Work dependent on a healthy body.

- social skills:The part of Age Work that allows kids to enjoy and benefit from being with others.

- communication:The part of Age Work that is language-based. School related abilities. The means by which "intelligence" is expressed.

OTHERS:A Consequence Area encompassing interaction with all others; family, neighbors, friends, etc. Failure to be accepted by Others is an objective criterion of *mis*/kidding.

AUTHORITY:A Consequence Area defined by a kid's relationships to people in charge, such as parents and teachers. Good/kidding requires acceptance of reasonable rules commensurate with mental age. Inability to accept reasonable rules is an objective criterion of *mis*/kidding.

LANGUAGE:Means of expressing ourselves.

- (W)ord (L)anguage:Things we say to kids to communicate to them.

- W/L Commands:Things we say to stop *mis*/kidding and to promote good/kidding.

- (A)ction (L)anguage:Actions or events that communicate to kids; language "spoken" by consequences.

A/L Consequences: Spontaneous or devised events that influence kidding.

- Deterrence: Use of an unpleasant (-) A/L Consequence, alone, to stop *mis*/kidding.

- Deflection: Use of a powerfully unpleasant (-) A/L Consequence to stop *mis*/kidding along with a mildly pleasant (+) A/L Consequence to encourage good/kidding.

- Diversion: Use of a mildly unpleasant (-) A/L Consequence to dissuade *mis*/kidding along with a powerfully pleasant (+) A/L Consequence to encourage good/kidding.

- Drawing: Use of a compelling pleasant (+) A/L Consequence, alone, to create motivation for good/kidding.

PARENTS: Adults who assume the HoNoR Role to grow kids into peers.

HoNoR Role: A model parents can use to raise kids, consisting of Honesty, Nurturance and Responsibility.

- Honesty: Keeping Word Language commands consistent with Action Language consequences.

- Nurturance: A supportive relationship between a kid and an adult comprised of love and affection. A powerful source of motivation for changing *mis*/kidding into good/kidding.

- Love: A series of acts that helps kids grow toward adulthood. It's "being there when it counts" and, as a heritage, is never contingent on good/kidding.

- Affection:A demonstration of liking and acceptance which can be made contingent upon good/kidding and offered as a reward.

- Superaffection: Things loved ones do to demonstrate liking and acceptance. The most powerful Action Language consequence (reward) for promoting good/kidding.

- Responsibility: The attribute that distinguishes kids from adults. When kids accept responsibility for the consequences of all their acts, they are adults.

PROFESSIONALS: People with special knowledge about kids and kidding who can help parents with *mis*/kidding: Physicians, Psychologists and Educators.

- Physician: A professional who examines and treats physical problems by doing lab tests, prescribing medicines, doing surgery or hospitalizing kids.

- Psychologist: A professional who can measure intelligence and assess emotion using standardized psychological tests and who can provide counseling and psychotherapy.

- Educator: A professional primarily concerned with academic performance and who has access to special schools and curriculae.

IDIOCIES: Fallacious beliefs that terrorize parents, creating guilt and eroding control over kids.

- Permissive idiocy: The belief that kids have the right to do whatever they please and that the world must adjust to their *mis*/kidding.

- Protective idiocy: The belief that kids are too frail to accept the consequences of their acts and too dumb to learn from them.

- Professional idiocy: The belief that professionals know the truth about everything and that only they are qualified to decide if, when or how *mis*/kidding should be managed.

Part One

Recognizing and Defining Misbehavior in Kids

The following three chapters present the diagnostic phase of the *MIS*/KIDDING process.

Here's how you decide:

- Is your kid's behavior worth doing anything about?
- Do you have time to develop a strategy to manage it, or do you need to stop it right away?
- Will you need professional help to control it?

CHAPTER ONE

Mis/kidding: The Kidding To Recognize

Mis/kidding is the "dark side" of the kidding force. It slows down or stops the process of growth and can even kill a kid. The constructive side of the force is good/kidding and is the path kids take to reach adulthood. Before I show you an easy way to identify *mis*/kidding, let's look at some examples of the two sides of kidding.

Kidding: Good/kidding and Mis/kidding At Various Ages

<u>Babies</u> cry, sleep and eat. At first, their kidding has a rhythm independent of their caretakers. The babies' needs determine the rhythm. Too long a wait between feedings, too little milk, or a stick with a diaper pin and babies cry. Whenever the cause of crying is obvious and can be controlled, we consider this "normal."

When babies begin to smile after feeding, coo at their parents and eagerly follow them with their eyes, this good/kidding bonds them to their parents and creates mutual enjoyment.

When babies cry too much, eat too much or too little, or otherwise do poorly, we recognize this as *mis*/kidding. Someone, usually the doctor or nurse in the hospital, must determine the cause of this *mis*/kidding and correct it.

<u>Later in infancy</u>, babies become more conscious of the world and develop desires. These include eating, sleeping and staying dry - all reasonable kidding.

When babies sleep through the night without waking their parents to eat, or sleep in spite of a wet diaper, that's good/kidding.

Babies' desires may also include refusing to give up the bottle, touching open flames, and rubbing spaghetti in their hair. These are all easily recognized forms of *mis*/kidding.

Toddlerhood is a time when kids explore the world. Testing rules and limits is usual and, within certain bounds, is considered "normal" kidding.

Developing better coordination, putting words into longer sentences, and the appearance of cooperative play with other kids are examples of good/kidding in toddlerhood.

Testing rules in toddlerhood becomes obvious *mis*/kidding when toddlers hit their baby brothers on the head with bottles, bite their nursery school teachers, or write on walls with lipstick.

The school years are a time for academic achievement, the making of friends, and heightened awareness of rules extending beyond the family. These are examples of good/kidding.

Underachievement in school, difficulty making or keeping friends, and the breaking of rules are easily recognized types of *mis*/kidding seen during the school years.

Adolescence is a transition period during which "kids" become adults. Education prepares kids for careers. Friendships develop into deeper relationships, and kids develop and follow their own working sets of rules and obligations. When they have achieved these goals and are ready to accept all the consequences of their acts, this good/kidding defines kids as adults.

Obvious examples of adolescent *mis*/kidding include drug abuse, unwanted pregnancy and attempted suicide. Failure to become adult-like, in all its varied ways, is the *mis*/kidding of adolescence.

Look at this list of *mis*/kidding:

- A baby crying for a bottle at night
- Overeating and under eating
- Refusing to give up the bottle
- Playing with fire
- Smearing spaghetti in hair
- Hitting brother on the head with a bottle
- Biting the teachers
- Writing on walls with lipstick
- Failing in school

- Not making friends
- Breaking rules of courtesy
- Drug abuse
- Unwanted pregnancy
- Attempting suicide

We recognize each of these as *mis*/kidding and know each must be controlled. Intuitively, we also know that some of these kinds of *mis*/kidding are more serious than others. In the next chapter, we'll see how to rank them by their seriousness. For now, let's ask how we know they're *mis*/kidding. The answer is we recognize *mis*/kidding by looking at its effects. At any stage of development, we look at the **consequences** of kidding to decide if it's *mis*/kidding.

Kidding can affect three areas of life. They're always the same. I call them the **CONSEQUENCE AREAS**:

Measures of Mis/kidding: The Consequence Areas

Reviewing our list of examples of *mis*/kidding in infancy, toddlerhood, the school years and adolescence reveals that at each stage we judge the effects of kidding on:

1. **AGE WORK**: This is kid's developmental (or age-related) growth. *Mis*/kidding is not achieving it.

2. **OTHERS**: *Mis*/kidding is not getting along with others, such that they consistently object to or complain about it.

3. **AUTHORITY**: *Mis*/kidding is breaking reasonable rules.

Kidding that interferes with one or more of these Consequence Areas is *mis*/kidding and may need to be shaped or controlled. In each example of *mis*/kidding listed above, **consequences** are affecting **AGE WORK, OTHERS** or **AUTHORITY**. Thus they may demand a response by an adult. I say they may demand a response because some forms of *mis*/kidding can be safely ignored.

Let's look at how we use these criteria to recognize *mis*/kidding.

AGE WORK: (Failing to Achieve at an age-appropriate level)

Age Work is the first and most important Consequence Area to examine to identify *mis*/kidding. That's because it's the foundation on which kids build their relationships to **Others** and to **Authority** persons. It's the most critical Consequence Area because within it lie all of the physical and mental handicaps **that take away kids' choice-making**. Fortunately, Age Work is the easiest area for parents to judge. Professionals have given us very precise criteria for what's "normal" and what's "abnormal" for every age. Age Work is the most objective of the Consequence Areas and many of its components are innate.

Let's take a look at the Consequence Area of Age Work. It's comprised of three ability areas:

The Three Ability Areas of Age Work

Age Work requires competence in three ability areas:

- **Physical** abilities - body control
- **Social** abilities - benefiting from interaction with others
- **Communication** abilities - language skills, including academic and intellectual abilities

Physical abilities, or body control, includes the development of normal muscle strength, tone and coordination for large and small muscles. Professionals divide these abilities into "fine" and "gross" *motor* skills. Though failure to progress normally in physical ability is often due to medical conditions, some delays in this area can be traced to poor choice-making by kids. I'll show you some examples soon. Normal physical ability for one age may be abnormal for another age.

Social abilities are the personal skills kids need at each age to learn from and enjoy the presence of others and to acquire self-esteem and self-confidence. They include ability to cope with the "stress" of rules and to compromise with others to attain mutual goals. To display adequate social abilities, kids must successfully find a middle ground between their wildest desires and society's strict rules. Kids' abilities to do this "normally" improve with age. The bounds of "normal" social ability are well defined by Professionals, but change slowly as society changes its values.

The social component of AGE WORK is an inward look at kids' skill development. It should not be confused with the outwardly directed Consequence Area of OTHERS' reactions to kids, which is explained below.

Communication skills, or language-related abilities, include all the skills kids use to make others aware of their thoughts and desires and which allow kids to understand the thoughts and desires of others. Academic skills are language-related abilities and are a part of *communication* skills. It's through language that intelligence is expressed.

Testing Kidding Against AGE WORK To Identify Mis/kidding

Kidding By Infants: How Age Work Defines Babies' *mis*/kidding

Normal six-month-old babies can sleep through the night without eating. They sit briefly without support and coo at their parents. A baby who fails to achieve these milestones is *mis*/kidding within the Consequence Area of Age Work:

ABILITY AREA OF *AGE WORK*	EXPECTED *AGE WORK*	OBSERVED *MIS*/KIDDING
Physical	Sits alone briefly	Doesn't sit at all
Social	Sleeps through night	Cries all night
Communication	Coos at parents	Doesn't vocalize

Kidding By Toddlers: How Age Work Defines Mis/kidding

Toddlers are expected to walk and climb well. They must also be able to understand and follow one or two commands. They should be able to play near or with other kids, and for the most part, peacefully. When a toddler can only crawl, seems unaware of or is unable to comprehend commands, or stays in a corner crying and sucking its thumb to the exclusion of other activities, it is *mis*/kidding in the area of **Age Work**:

Ability Area of *AGE WORK*	Expected *AGE WORK*	Observed *MIS*/KIDDING
Physical	Walks and climbs	Only crawls or lies on floor
Social	Plays near or with other kids	Sits in a corner sucks thumb or cries
Communication	Follows one or two commands	Seems unaware of commands

Kidding By Elementary Schoolers: AGE WORK Defines Mis/kidding

Elementary schoolers are expected to go to school unless they are ill. They're expected to be able to use a pencil, attend to their bathroom needs and communicate with their teachers. If an elementary schooler can't hold a pencil, wets or soils his pants repeatedly or doesn't speak to his teachers, he's *mis*/kidding in the area of Age Work. Whenever kidding fails to reach the expected ("normal") Age Work for that age or phase, it's *mis*/kidding:

Ability Area of *AGE WORK*	Expected *AGE WORK*	Observed *MIS*/KIDDING
Physical	Can hold and use a pencil	Can't hold or use a pencil
Social	Uses bathroom properly	Wets or soils clothes
Communication	Speaks with teacher	Doesn't speak with teacher

Kidding By an Adolescent: Age Work Defines Mis/kidding

Adolescents are expected to keep friendships (without the help of drunk driving). They should be able to participate in physical education activities at school and maintain their grades in the range of their abilities. Losing friends, deteriorating stamina or coordination, or suddenly falling grades are examples of *mis*/kidding in the Age Work of adolescence:

Ability Area of *AGE WORK*	Expected *AGE WORK*	Observed *MIS*/KIDDING
Physical	Adequate stamina and coordination	Deteriorating physical ability
Social	Keeping and enlarging friendships	Losing friends; drunk driving
Communication	Maintaining grades	Failing grades

Although the Consequence Area of **Age Work** is the most important and critical test for the presence of *mis*/kidding, most kids will "pass" the test. That is, they will be achieving normally in physical, social and communication development. The importance of passing the test of Age Work is that *mis*/kidding defined by the remaining Consequence Areas of

Others and Authority is <u>always under kids' control</u>. The *mis*/kidding is therefore potentially under parents' control. More about this later.

The next "test" is within the Consequence Area of **OTHERS**. The reaction of OTHER people to kids is less objective than Age Work, since it's "in the eyes of the beholder." Sometimes, though, simply counting the number of complaints from teachers, neighbors, friends and even policemen will give a very objective picture of *mis*/kidding!

Let's look at the Consequence Area of **OTHERS** and how it's used to recognize *mis*/kidding.

OTHERS: (Disturbing those around you)

How kids get along with those around them is not only determined by the quality of their behavior, but also by Others' reactions to it. Parents must make their own observations as they take note of OTHERS' reactions to their kids.

Testing Kidding Against OTHERS To Recognize Mis/kidding

Revisiting Kidding By Babies- Recognizing Mis/kidding By Its Effect On OTHERS:

Though some parents may not mind babies crying through the night to be fed or held, visitors to their home may feel otherwise. When baby-sitters, relatives, or the grandparents sleep over, objections are likely to be raised. Whether or not the parents see this behavior as unacceptable for their baby, the effect of the kidding on OTHERS is decided <u>by the Others</u>. If Others decide baby crying all night is unacceptable, and they must continue to stay with the parents, the kidding becomes *mis*/kidding. Parents who accept babies crying all night can prevent this from becoming *mis*/kidding only by <u>avoiding ill consequences to Others.</u> When Others are in the picture, *they* decide whether the criterion of complaints by Others has been met. Others can decide, too, that babies crying all night do not distress them.

Revisiting Kidding In Toddlerhood- Recognizing Mis/kidding By Its Effect On OTHERS:

In our example of the toddler who becomes mute in nursery school and begins to withdraw and suck his thumb, the teacher and classmates may view this kidding, at least for a while, as normal or acceptable. If other kids in the class begin to imitate this kidding, or begin to tease the mute kid, keeping control of the class or getting work done will be difficult. If the consequence of the kidding to Others is unacceptable to either the teacher or to others, the kidding becomes *mis*/kidding.

Revisiting Mis/kidding In An Elementary Schooler- Recognizing Mis/kidding By Its Effect On OTHERS:

The elementary schooler who tantrums on the floor at home when the school bus comes, but whose parents accept this kidding, has avoided an ill effect in the Consequence Area of OTHERS (It's the parents who'll have problems with the school). For these parents, this behavior is just kidding. Since there are no effects on Others, this kid's behavior does not qualify as *mis*/kidding. On the other hand, if the parents don't accept this kidding, it becomes *mis*/kidding.

Revisiting Mis/kidding In Adolescence- Effects on OTHERS:

The adolescent who drinks and drives intoxicated very much affects OTHERS. Both those put at risk by such actions, and those who enforce the law, are affected by the kidding. In this example, these consequences for Others are independent of parents and define the kidding as *mis*/kidding.

If kids have "passed the test" of **AGE WORK**, but are *mis*/kidding within the area of Others, they are always making a choice for *mis*/kidding. That is, there is no innate reason for the *mis*/kidding.

The third and last Consequence Area of kidding that defines *mis*/kidding is **AUTHORITY**. This is certainly the most subjective of the Consequence Areas. What is unruly or undisciplined *mis*/kidding for some parents is merely acceptable kidding or even praiseworthy good/kidding for others. So long as AGE WORK and OTHERS are unaffected, judgments within the area of AUTHORITY are truly "in the eye of the beholder."

AUTHORITY (Breaking reasonable rules)

As kids become aware of the differences between themselves and other people, their desires come more into conflict with the expectations of their caretakers. At each age, they must somehow reach a balance between satisfying their most urgent desires and acting within limits set by those in Authority around them.

When kids try to satisfy desires that extend beyond acceptable limits, the *consequence* is a threat to AUTHORITY. Threatened AUTHORITY relationships are a final measure of *mis*/kidding.

Developing normal AUTHORITY relationships, like relating well to OTHERS, requires two things: a healthy enough brain to be able to make choices and motivation to make right choices. In Chapter Three we'll see that passing the test of AGE WORK means kids' brains are healthy. We'll see that when kids pass the test of AGE WORK, but fail the subsequent tests of OTHERS or AUTHORITY, it means they're making bad choices.

A Final Visit To Kidding In Babies- Recognizing Mis/kidding By Its Effect On AUTHORITY:

It's not unusual for six month old babies to awaken at night and cry until they're held or fed. If this pattern continues, it can become *mis*/kidding. Babies learn to cry to be held. Their desires for attention and stimulation can lead them to choose to cry until parents are compelled to hold them. A consequence of such kidding is that parents break their (unspoken) rule that nighttime is for sleeping. This becomes *mis*/kidding only if the parents have a rule that nighttime is for sleeping! In some homes, nighttime is for feeding babies. Since in those homes, babies crying have no impact on AUTHORITY (and I'm not there as an OTHER!), there is no *mis*/kidding.

A Final Visit To Kidding By Toddlers- How Its Effect On AUTHORITY Defines Mis/kidding:

Toddlers occasionally resort to biting their caretakers and other kids. This usually occurs during temper tantrums and is not otherwise frequently seen. Sometimes temper tantrums and biting are kids' preferred responses to the setting of limits. When this becomes a pattern of response to AUTHORITY, either the parents' or the teachers', it becomes *mis*/kidding.

I've met parents who accept being bitten by their kids. If they are their kids' sole targets and do not consider their AUTHORITY relationship threatened, there is no *mis*/kidding. When their kids bite OTHERS (whether in AUTHORITY or not), *mis*/kidding is defined.

A Final Visit To Kidding By Elementary Schoolers- How Its Effect On AUTHORITY Defines Mis/kidding:

Elementary schoolers may refuse to go to school each morning by choosing to lie on the floor and shriek as the bus comes. Some parents feel obliged to allow their kids to stay home. If the parents have a rule that kids must go to school each day except for illness, and their kids are not ill, this is *mis*/kidding. If the parents don't have a rule that healthy kids must go to school, there's no threat to their AUTHORITY, and they will recognize no *mis*/kidding.

A Final Visit To Kidding In Adolescence- Recognizing Mis/kidding By Its Effect On AUTHORITY:

Adolescents often party and sometimes drink and drive. If their parents have made it clear they're not to drink alcohol if they're planning to drive, then overruling their parents' AUTHORITY defines *mis*/kidding. If the parents have no such rule, but the hosts of the party do, breaking their rule defines *mis*/kidding. If neither the parents nor the hosts have the rule, but kids are arrested by the police, breaking the AUTHORITY of the law defines *mis*/kidding. In each case, countermanding someone's AUTHORITY by breaking reasonable rules defines *mis*/kidding.

Some parents and some hosts don't have rules for drinking and driving. For them, as long as no police are involved, their kids are only kidding.

Applying the test of AUTHORITY to identify *mis*/kidding is to use the most personal (subjective) of the Consequence Areas. When we use the Consequence Area of OTHERS, we receive outside (more objective) opinions from others and since we as parents are a part of "Others" we also make personal, subjective judgments of our own. Measuring kidding against AGE WORK is most objective, since professionals have measured and defined all the components of AGE WORK in detail.

Here's an easy way to visualize the Consequence Areas, from the most innate and objective area of AGE WORK to the most volitional and subjective area, AUTHORITY.

Remember, it's important to identify *mis*/kidding because it slows down or stops kids from reaching adulthood and because no one has enough energy to control all kidding. We identify *mis*/kidding by applying the "tests" of the Consequence Areas. Let's review what we've learned.

Using The Consequence Areas Of AGE WORK, OTHERS And AUTHORITY to Identify Mis/kidding

When you try to decide if kidding is really *mis*/kidding, put the kidding to the test by asking whether it sets back or even stops progress in any of the three Consequence Areas:

AGE WORK: See if the kidding is setting back or preventing progress in **any** of the three ability areas of AGE WORK (*physical, social,* and *communication*). If it is, you've identified *mis*/kidding.

OTHERS: Whether or not your authority is affected, ask (or listen, for you may be told) whether Others are having a problem with the kidding. If they are, the kidding is *mis*/kidding.

AUTHORITY: As a parent, you'll know if your Authority is set back. If so, you've got *mis*/kidding. If anyone else's reasonable rules are threatened, you've also got *mis*/kidding.

The *Consequence Areas*

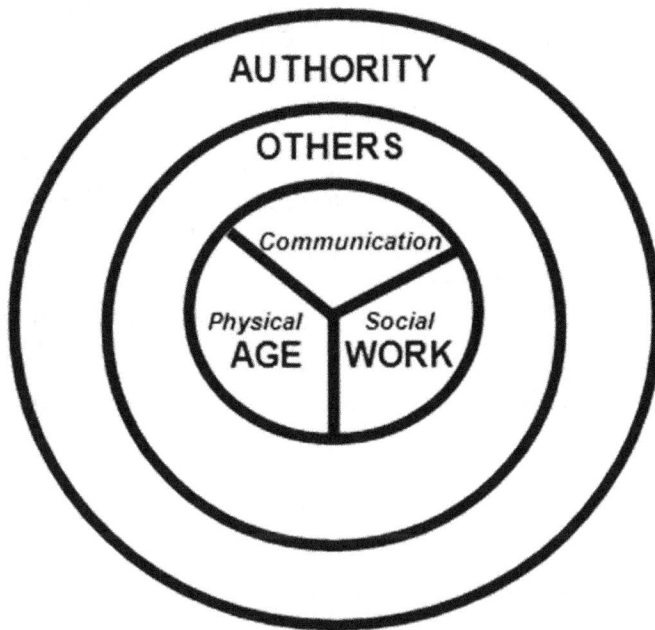

AUTHORITY

OTHERS

Communication

Physical
AGE

Social
WORK

It's not necessary to determine the cause of *mis*/kidding to be sure it is *mis*/kidding. Whether a cause is a *physical condition* or a *bad choice* by a kid, it is still *mis*/kidding and it may need to be shaped or controlled. In using this book, you don't have to know what "normal" AGE WORK is for every kid. Normal AGE WORK is presented for each age or phase in **APPENDIX I**. As you might guess, when *mis*/kidding affects AGE WORK, the cause can be very serious. It's in the area of Age Work that *mis*/kidding most often requires the help of an expert. Soon I'll show you how to tell when you need a Professional and which one.

Before you learn how to determine the **seriousness** of *mis*/kidding, once you've identified it, let's look at one last exaggerated example of kidding. People who use only intuition to identify *mis*/kidding might have trouble classifying it. You, of course, armed with your knowledge of the three Consequence Areas, will have no problem with it!

The Case of a Kid Who Sleeps On His Head

A father finishes work late and sneaks into the room of his three-year-old son at 2 AM. He sees his son leaning on his head, feet propped against the wall, fast asleep! Dad observes for thirty minutes, but can see no apparent ill effects.

He's confused and returns to his own bed to ponder this strange behavior. He sneaks back at 6 AM and finds his son sleeping "normally" on his side.

The next night, his curiosity aroused, Dad returns to his son's room. Once again at 2 AM his son is sleeping on his head, feet propped against the wall. This time, Dad remains until 6 AM, when his son slides onto his side, still fast asleep, and remains in that position till 8 AM. He then awakens as usual for nursery school.

Dad notices his son is neither tired nor irritable. The boy eats well. He goes off to nursery school with his usual friends. The teacher reports no problems. Mom notices nothing out of the ordinary. Dad, who has yet to read *MIS*/KIDDING, calls Dr. Davick to find out whether this is a problem, but the doctor is out. So father, who happens to be your neighbor, consults you instead. Using the three Consequence Areas, your notes look like this:

AGE WORK: No effect on *physical, social* or *communication* skills

OTHERS: No effect on Others

AUTHORITY: No reasonable rules broken

You conclude the boy is only kidding. His father goes home pacified. His son may still be sleeping on his head between the hours of 2 AM and 6 AM, but who cares? Perhaps the boy's wife, in years to come, will complain as an Other and thus define "marital" *mis*/kidding, but that's for another book!

Your neighbor may wake up one night wondering why his son sleeps on his head. If he wishes to engage in the Professional Idiocy and consult an expert about this behavior, he will surely find one to assess this *non-problem*. It may be an expensive, time-consuming and anxiety-provoking experience.

Unfortunately, parents often squander a lot of money and energy struggling with kidding rather than focusing on *mis*/kidding.

Now that you can identify *mis*/kidding, you must learn how to grade its *severity*. Which *mis*/kidding must be dealt with *soonest,* which is most *dangerous,* which (if any) can be *ignored?*

In Summary:

To Recognize *Mis*/kidding, check kidding against the **Consequence Areas-**

1. Check the three skill areas of AGE WORK.

•Is the kid failing to achieve the *physical* development expected for that age? Is the kid *physically* threatened by the kidding?

•Is the kid failing to benefit from *social* interactions as expected for that age? Are *social* interactions threatened by the kidding?

•Are the kid's <u>observed</u> *communication* skills falling below the level expected for that age? Is mental achievement threatened by the kidding?

2. Check if the kidding creates threats to or complaints from **OTHERS**, including yourself.

3. Check if the kidding threatens someone's **AUTHORITY**.

If the answer to any of these questions is "yes", you've identified *mis*/kidding.

CHAPTER TWO

Mid/kidding: The Mis/kidding To Redirect

Now that you can recognize *mis*/kidding by its effects on the Consequence Areas, you need to know how much time you have to control or correct it. You do this by judging the severity of the *mis*/kidding.

Mis/kidding can be judged by (1) the feelings or emotions it *evokes* in the observer (that is, *you*), and (2) by its *effects* on you, the kid and others. When you weigh *mis*/kidding by your emotions, you're using a *subjective* test. This means you're feeling the emotions and you're making the judgment. Think about the last time you watched kids misbehaving. Depending on how impudent they were, you probably experienced one or more of the emotions on this list:

Annoyance

Confusion

Anxiety

Anger

FEAR

When you judge the effects or *consequences* of *mis*/kidding, you're anticipating a bad outcome for you, the kid, or others. In contrast to gauging *mis*/kidding subjectively by your emotions, using this more objective test of Consequence Areas, means that others beside yourself may play a part in judging the impact your kid's actions.

The best way to judge the severity of *mis*/kidding, and the time you can take to solve the problem, is to combine <u>both</u> *subjective* and *objective* measures.

I'll show you how to do this a little later in the chapter. First, let's take a closer look at the subjective criterion of emotions.

Look at a rearranged list of the *mis*/kidding we examined in Chapter One. In columns alongside the list I've indicated the *severity* and the reactions or *emotions* evoked in an observer of the *mis*/kidding. The *emotions* I've listed are the subjective criteria. It's not important that you feel exactly what I feel. What is important is that you begin to rank your feelings into one of three categories: (1) *mild* or "cool" reactions, where the kidding is "annoying" or "trivial" (2) *Moderate* or "Warm" reactions, like "Confusion", "Anxiety" or "Anger', and (3) *SEVERE* or "HOT" reactions, like "FEAR." Later in this chapter, after you've seen how to use your emotional response to judge the severity of *mis*/kidding, I'll show you how to combine these subjective criteria with the more objective Consequence Areas to fully define *mis*/kidding.

Severity	Examples Of *Mis*/kidding	Emotion Felt By Observer
VERY SEVERE **"HOT"**	**Toddler playing with fire** **Adolescent attempting suicide** **Toddler hitting brother with a bottle** **Elementary schooler abusing drugs** **Adolescent in danger of unwanted pregnancy**	*FEAR*
More Severe	**A baby crying round the clock** **Failing in school** **Not making friends and losing old ones** **Overeating and under eating**	*Anxiety*
Moderate "Warm"	**Biting the nursery school teacher** **Writing on walls with lipstick** **Smearing spaghetti in hair** **Being discourteous**	*Anger*
Less Severe	**Refusing to give up bottle at 2 years age** **Baby crying for a bottle at night**	*Confusion*
mild "cool"	**Refusing to hug or kiss Mommy** **Not finishing a meal** **Saying, "You're a bad Mommy or Daddy."**	annoyance

Using the Subjective Criteria For *Mis*/kidding: *KILLER*/kidding, *Mid*/kidding and mini/kidding

In the list above, see how **SEVERE** *mis*/kidding is associated with **FEAR**, a "HOT" emotional response in the observer. I call **SEVERE** *mis*/kidding, that causes **FEAR**, or a "HOT" emotional response in the observer, **KILLER/kidding**, because it threatens major injury or death to kids or others in the short-term. *KILLER*/kidding must be "chilled" **immediately**, with **overwhelming force**, if necessary. While injury or death are imminent, time cannot be taken to find out the reasons for its occurrence.

Moderate mis/kidding is associated with "Warm" emotional responses in the observer, like *Anxiety,* *Anger* or *Confusion*. I call Moderate *mis*/kidding, *Mid*/kidding. *Mid*/kidding needs to be controlled because it can cause injury or death to kids or others over the long-term. *Mid*/kidding allows time to discover causes and to develop strategies for its control.

Mild mis/kidding, which causes only "cool" emotional responses in the observer, like annoyance, I call *mini*/kidding. *Mini*/kidding, unless it continues for a very long time, cannot cause harm to kids or others. *Mini*/kidding can safely be ignored.

To structure your thinking about your emotional responses when you encounter *mis*/kidding, and to make it easier to use these criteria when you measure the "temperature" of *mis*/kidding, I've assigned "degrees" to each category of emotion:

Category	Emotional Response	Designated "Degrees"
HOT (SEVERE)	*FEAR*	3 degrees
Warm (Moderate)	*Anxiety, Anger or Confusion*	2 degrees
Cool (mild)	*annoyance*	1 degree

Parents are remarkably consistent in describing their feelings about different types of *mis*/kidding. Though the greatest diversity of emotions is described within the category of *Mid*/kidding (where one observer may be anxious while another is merely confused), few people disagree enough on the intensity of their reactions to differ on a whole category of *mis*/kidding.

We may be even more certain of the "temperature" of *mis*/kidding if we use the more *objective* Consequence Areas along with our subjective feelings. Used together, the subjective and objective criteria accurately measure the intensity of *mis*/kidding. When we develop plans to control *mis*/kidding, we'll check the Consequence Areas to be sure our solution to the *mis*/kidding problem has worked. As soon as the objective criteria are obliterated, the *mis*/kidding is gone and the problem is "solved."

Using Objective Criteria for *Mis*/kidding: Assigning Degrees to The Consequence Areas

Just as it's possible to label the intensity of the "heat" of our subjective emotional reactions to *mis*/kidding, we can quantify the effects of *mis*/kidding on the more objective Consequence Areas.

AGE WORK: You already know that the skill areas of *physical, social* and *communication* have a large innate component. This means that *mis*/kidding affecting any of these areas could be hereditary or due to a handicap or an illness. *Mis*/kidding in any of these areas may not be under kids' control, or yours either.

Because AGE WORK is the most objectively judged of the Consequence Areas, and because problems within it are the most potentially serious, I have assigned *each* skill area one degree of intensity. When all three skill areas of AGE WORK are affected by *mis*/kidding, 3 degrees are derived.

OTHERS: There are two groups of OTHERS that can be affected by *mis*/kidding; (1) you, and (2) everybody else! I've assigned 1 degree to you and 1 degree to everybody else. When both You and Others beside you are affected by *mis*/kidding, the Consequence Area of OTHERS can generate 2 degrees.

AUTHORITY: The effect of *mis*/kidding on your AUTHORITY defines the least objective of the

The *Consequence Areas*

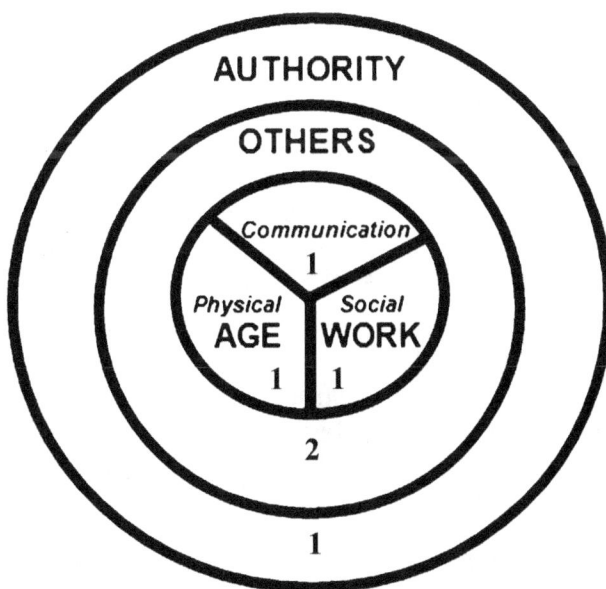

Consequence Areas. For this reason, and because the effects of *mis*/kidding on OTHERS are already accounted for, I've assigned this entire Consequence

Area 1 degree of "heat." Here's a diagram you've seen before. The objective Consequence Areas are now shown with the "degrees" each can generate:

Below is a summary of the scoring system for ranking the severity of *mis*/kidding. To see how it's applied to real-life situations, read on:

Subjective Criteria (Your Emotional Response)	Intensity ("Heat")	Objective Criteria The Consequence Areas	Intensity ("Heat")
FEAR ("HOT") =	3 degrees	AGE WORK *Physical* = *Social* = Communication = Possible Total =	1 degree 1 degree 1 degree 3 degrees
Anger Anxiety ("*Warm*") = Confusion	2 degrees	OTHERS You = Others = Possible Total =	1 degree 1 degree 2 degrees
annoyance ("cool") =	1 degree	AUTHORITY =	1 degree

Using Subjective WITH Objective Criteria to Define Severity: Scoring the Effects of *Mis*/kidding (Or How "Hot" The Problem)

There's a reason why people feel varying degrees of emotional response ranging from mere annoyance, through Confusion, Anger and Anxiety, to outright FEAR when they encounter different gradations of *mis*/kidding. It's because the "hotter" the *mis*/kidding becomes, the more severe are its consequences. More severe consequences disturb us more when we recognize them. Whenever we observe *mis*/kidding, we subconsciously gauge objective and subjective "degrees." The metering system I've shown you makes this a more conscious process. The higher the degrees, the "hotter" and more destructive the consequences of the *mis*/kidding. The lower the degrees, the "cooler" the *mis*/kidding and the longer it will take to "burn" kids or others. If the degrees are low enough, it can never burn anyone and can be safely ignored.

Here's a "thermometer" for *mis*/kidding. The degrees listed on the left side of the thermometer are *combined subjective* and *objective* criteria for any type of *mis*/kidding. Focus on the ranges of degrees for ***KILLER***/kidding,

Mid/kidding and *mini*/kidding. They'll become very familiar to you as we use them to look at examples of *mis*/kidding on the next few pages.

Degrees Of *Mis*/kidding

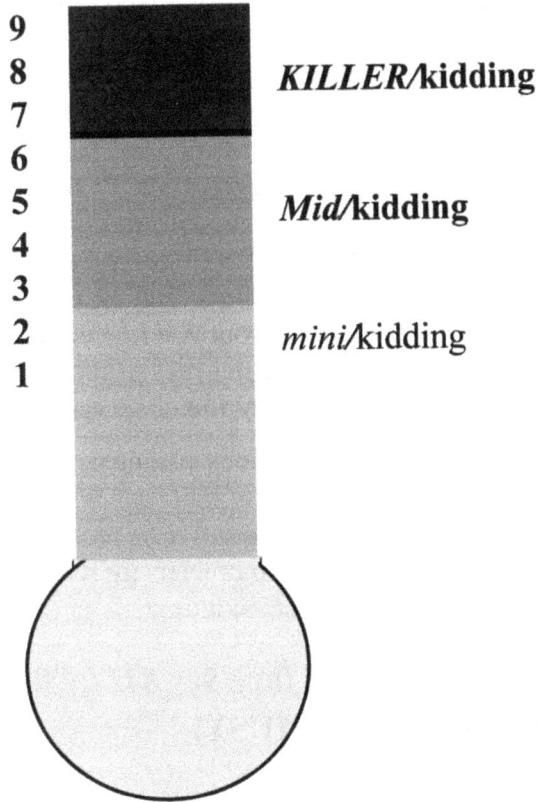

9
8   **KILLER/kidding**
7

6
5   ***Mid*/kidding**
4

3
2   *mini*/kidding
1

KILLER/kidding: Turn Down the Heat Immediately!

When you see a "temperature" of **7 thru 9,** you've got **KILLER/kidding**. Many parents don't recognize *KILLER*/kidding if kids' lives are not in immediate *physical* danger. One of the benefits of the *mis*/kidding thermometer is that by using it to gauge *mis*/kidding, you can identify "hot" problems that will lead to severe outcomes *before* kids or others around them are physically threatened.

In situations where kids may be provoked into attempted suicide, for example, the "temperature" of the *mis*/kidding will rise into the *KILLER*/kidding range long before any physical threat is seen. This thermometer identifies lethal problems *early*.

The appropriate response to *KILLER/kidding* is always **direct intervention** to diminish it to a lower level of *mis*/kidding. Such intervention is not negotiable.

When life or limb are threatened, **overwhelming force may be necessary**. As you read on, I'll show you how *KILLER*/kidding can be "cooled" down to *Mid*/kidding or *mini*/kidding.

Using the *Mis*/kidding Thermometer to Identify *KILLER*/kidding

KILLER/kidding degrees of **7 thru 9** are usually derived from objective effects on the three skill areas of AGE WORK (3 degrees), plus both components of OTHERS (2 degrees), plus at least a "Warm" emotional (subjective) reaction to the *Mis*/kidding (another 2 degrees or more). Other combinations are possible, but *KILLER*/kidding is always present when the total temperature reaches **7 degrees** or more. **This is so even if FEAR is not the emotion experienced by the observer.**

Here are some obvious examples of *KILLER*/kidding. In each case, the *mis*/kidding threatens to snuff out a kid's life. These are the kinds of *KILLER*/kidding parents intuitively recognize without a scoring system. Later, we'll use the thermometer to recognize more subtle, but equally dangerous forms of *KILLER*/kidding.

Temperatures Of 7 thru 9 = *KILLER*/kidding: STOP IT HOWEVER YOU MUST!

Example Of *KILLER/kidding*	*Objective* Degrees	*Subjective* Degrees	Total
A baby choking and blue	AGE WORK = 3 Life-threat to all three *skill areas* OTHERS = 2 You lose baby Others in family lose baby	HOT *(FEAR)* = 3	8 degrees

In this situation, most parents are frightened. This "HOT" reaction registers 3 degrees. Since the baby could die, all 3 skill areas of AGE WORK would be affected and would generate another 3 degrees. All the OTHERS (you, and <u>everybody else</u> relating to the baby would also be affected, yielding 2 more degrees. The *Mis*/kidding thermometer would read **8** degrees, identifying ***KILLER*/kidding**.

Here are some similar examples of *KILLER*/kidding in other age ranges:

Example Of *KILLER/kidding*	Objective Degrees	Subjective Degrees	Total
A toddler jumping in front of a car	<u>AGE WORK</u> =3 Life-threat to all <u>three</u> *skill areas* <u>OTHERS</u> =2 <u>You</u> lose toddler <u>Others</u> in family lose toddler	HOT *(FEAR)* =3	8 degrees

Examples Of *KILLER/kidding*	Objective Degrees	Subjective Degrees	Total
A three year old playing on the sill of an open third-story window	<u>AGE WORK</u> = 3 Life threat to all <u>three</u> *skill areas* <u>OTHERS</u> = 2 <u>You</u> lose the kid Others in family lose the kid	HOT *(FEAR)* = 3	8 degrees

Examples Of *KILLER/kidding*	*Objective* Degrees	*Subjective* Degrees	Total
Attempted suicide by a teenager	AGE WORK =3 Life threat to all three *skill areas* OTHERS =2 You lose the kid Others in family lose the kid	HOT *(FEAR)* =3	8 degrees

The three examples above are "HOT", scary scenarios, each registering 3 subjective degrees. Threats to all three skill areas of AGE WORK in each case generate 3 more degrees. Again, you and the Others may lose the kids, adding 2 more degrees in each instance. For each situation, a total of **8** degrees defines ***KILLER*/kidding**.

Small differences within the subjective and objective areas, that is, between emotional responses you *feel* and effects you can *see*, rarely diminish the "heat" of "*KILLER*/kidding. For example, people who react to a suicide attempt with *Anger* (2 degrees) rather than *FEAR* (3 degrees), usually see this act as a threat to their AUTHORITY (adding back another degree). Whenever the total "temperature" reaches or exceeds **7** degrees, you've got *KILLER*/kidding**.**

Now let's see how the *mis*/kidding thermometer identifies *KILLER*/kidding before there's a direct threat to life. Parents don't usually recognize these types of *KILLER*/kidding until they've become life-threatening situations:

Examples Of *KILLER/kidding*	*Objective* Degrees	*Subjective* Degrees	Total
A four year old bites anyone who approaches and mutilates himself; spoken language is limited to single words	AGE WORK =3 *Physical* *Social* *Communication* OTHERS =2 - Bites You - Bites Others AUTHORITY =1 - Breaking rules	*Warm (Anxiety)* =2	8 degrees

Examples Of *KILLER/kidding*	*Objective* Degrees	*Subjective* Degrees	Total
A fifteen year old losing friends, always tired, falling grades, stealing from you and from grandparents	AGE WORK =3 *Physical* *Social* *Communication* OTHERS =2 -Steals from _You_ -Steals from Others AUTHORITY =1 -Breaking rules	*Warm (Anxiety)* =2	8 degrees

Take the "*KILLER*" Out of *KILLER*/kidding: Focus On AGE WORK and Convert To *Mid*/kidding

In Chapter One you learned to identify *mis*/kidding, the first step toward controlling it. Now you know how to recognize *KILLER*/kidding by its degrees of intensity. If you look closely, you'll see that *KILLER*/kidding *always affects at least one <u>skill area</u> of AGE WORK*. This means there may be a serious underlying reason for the *mis*/kidding - one that could be innate and uncontrollable by the kid. The second step in controlling *mis*/kidding, and one which is taken before attempting to discover causes, is to convert the *KILLER*/kidding into *Mid*/kidding. Beginning with the affected skill areas of AGE WORK, and continuing with OTHERS (leaving AUTHORITY for last), "chill" the most threatening parts of the *KILLER*/kidding until its "temperature" falls below 7.

You must do this quickly and with whatever degree of force is necessary. If a kid is too big for you to control, you must get help. Once the *KILLER*/kidding is converted to *Mid*/kidding, you'll have time to develop a plan to correct or control it. Once I've shown you how this strategy is applied to the previous examples of *KILLER*/kidding, we'll look at the *mis*/kidding thermometer again as it's used to identify *Mid*/kidding and *mini*/kidding.

Converting *KILLER*/kidding To *Mid*/kidding

Here are the examples of *KILLER*/kidding you saw above. Each of them measures **8** degrees on the *mis*/kidding thermometer:

- A baby choking and blue
- A toddler jumping in front of a car
- A three year old playing in an open window
- Attempted suicide by a teenager
- A four year old biting everyone, mutilating himself and using only single words

In each situation, threats to AGE WORK contribute 3 degrees. For these examples, the fastest way to convert the *KILLER*/kidding to *Mid*/kidding is to remove the kid from physical danger. This "cools" the threat to AGE WORK and diminishes the "heat" by at least 3 degrees.

For the baby, clearing the airway, giving CPR and getting medical help preserve AGE WORK. When accomplished, these steps may bring the *mis*/kidding "temperature" to zero ("just" kidding). For the toddler, and the three year old, physically removing them from danger preserves AGE WORK. If they attempt to repeat the *mis*/kidding while they're being supervised, their parents may suspect problems within the communication area of AGE WORK (1 degree), perceive a threat to AUTHORITY (1 degree) and become ANGRY (2 degrees). The *mis*/kidding, now reading 4 degrees, has been converted to *Mid*/kidding because the kids have been removed from immediate danger and are supervised.

For the suicidal teenager and the 4 year old with bizarre and dangerous self-mutilation and biting, forceful removal from immediate peril is necessary. For most parents, this requires help from professionals, usually at a hospital. In the next chapter, I'll show you how to choose the right professional(s) for the job. In these last examples, hospitalization "chills" the *KILLER*/kidding enough to convert it to *Mid*/kidding and allows you time to develop a strategy for ultimate control.

Identifying *KILLER*/kidding and converting it to a lesser degree of *mis*/kidding saves kids' lives. No detailed understanding or complex calculation is required by a parent to achieve this. As in the first three examples above, taking the "*KILLER*" out of *KILLER*/kidding often leaves little or no *mis*/kidding behind. Sometimes, as in the last two examples, some *mis*/kidding remains.

When you convert *KILLER*/kidding to a lesser degree of *mis*/kidding, or when you encounter "cooler" levels of *mis*/kidding, the thermometer you've used before will distinguish *Mid*/kidding from *mini*/kidding. Remember that *Mid*/kidding can became *KILLER*/kidding if it's ignored too long. This is why we develop a plan to control *Mid*/kidding as soon as we've eliminated the *KILLER*/kidding. I'll tell you more about *mini*/kidding later. Let's use our "temperature" scale to define *Mid*/kidding.

Using the *Mis*/kidding Thermometer to Identify *Mid*/kidding

Mid/kidding produces **3, 4, 5,** or **6** "degrees" on the *Mis*/kidding scale. This is the *mis*/kidding with the widest range of diversity. Almost any combination of *Consequence Areas* (objective degrees) and emotional responses by the observer (subjective degrees) can add up to *Mid*/kidding.. Because *Mid*/kidding takes so many forms, the vast majority of our attention is devoted to its management. But don't despair! The process of redirecting *Mid*/kidding, which I'll teach you in Chapters Four and Five, is very easy to learn and use.

For now, let's focus on identifying *Mid*/kidding in the following examples:

(See chart on the next page.)

Temperatures of 3, 4, 5, or 6 = *Mid*/kidding: Plan to Redirect It

Example Of *Mid*/kidding	*Objective* Degrees	*Subjective* Degrees	Total
An infant turning blue in the face during a breath holding spell	AGE WORK =1 *Physical* OTHERS =1 -Threat to *You*	*Warm* *(Anxiety)* = 2	4 degrees
A toddler not walking at eighteen months	AGE WORK =1 *Physical*	*Warm* *(Anxiety)* =2	3 degrees
A preschooler refusing to separate from mother in nursery school	AGE WORK =1 *Social* OTHERS =1 -Disturbs others	*Cool* *(Annoying)* =1	3 degrees
A 5 year old smearing feces on a wall	AGE WORK =1 *Social* OTHERS =2 -*You* are offended -Others complain AUTHORITY =1	*Warm (Anger)* =2	6 degrees
An elementary schooler not learning to read	AGE WORK =1 *Communication* OTHERS =1	*Warm* *(Anxiety)* =2	4 degrees
Sudden onset of bed-wetting in a previously "dry" 8 year old	AGE WORK =1 *Physical* OTHERS =1 -*You*	*"Warm"* *(Confusion)* = 2	4 degrees
An adolescent lying to a parent	AGE WORK =1 *Social* OTHERS =1 -*You*, if parent AUTHORITY =1	*Warm (Anger)* =2	5 degrees

You can see how the effects of kidding on AGE WORK are easiest to judge, while effects on OTHERS and AUTHORITY are more open to differences of opinion. That's why *Mid*/kidding has a wider range of degrees than *KILLER*/kidding and *mini*/kidding.

You also see from these examples how most people will agree on the intensity of their emotional response, even though some might be *Angered* while others are *Confused* or *Anxious*.

We've just seen how, after recognizing *mis*/kidding, the second step toward its control is to convert any *KILLER*/kidding to *Mid*/kidding. What do we do with lesser degrees of *mis*/kidding that are neither *KILLER*/kidding nor even "warm" enough to have reached the level of *Mid*/kidding? Such *mis*/kidding, measuring only **1 or 2** degrees on the "thermometer", is *mini*/kidding.

Using the *Mis*/kidding Thermometer to Identify *mini*/kidding

Though kids are "out of control" when they're *mini*/kidding, the only Consequence Area affected by the kidding is the AUTHORITY of the observer (1 degree) and his or her possible feeling of annoyance (1 degree). If a "temperature" of more than 2 degrees is reached on the scale, such as a threat to AUTHORITY (1 degree) with Anger (2 degrees), the *mis*/kidding is no longer *mini*/kidding, but has reached the mild *Mid*/kidding range.

When an observer, even a parent, perceives a threat to AUTHORITY without consequences to the kid or anyone else, *it's best to ignore the mis/kidding.* Only when persistent *mini*/kidding creates enough "heat" to become *Mid*/kidding is it worth the time and effort to respond to it. Here are some examples of *mini*/kidding:

Temperatures of 1 or 2 = *mini*/kidding: Ignore It!

Examples Of *mini*/kidding	*Objective* Degrees	*Subjective* Degrees	Total
A toddler saying, "Daddy, I hate you," after being denied dessert.	AUTHORITY = 1	*"cool" (annoying)* = 1	2 degrees
An elementary schooler crying for Mommy after being put to bed	(no consequences)	*"cool" (annoying)* = 1	1 degree

Can We Really Ignore mini/kidding?

Mini/kidding is a very personal experience for an adult. After all, *no one else suffers any consequences*. Because grown-ups have only so much energy, it's best to avoid making rules for kids to follow if those rules aren't worth using energy to enforce. This is especially true if labor must first be spent converting *KILLER*/kidding or managing *Mid*/kidding. *Controlling mini*/kidding *is a luxury you can't afford!* I suggest you let *mini*/kidding go away by itself.

Here are some rules I've seen parents make to control *mis*/kidding. If only 1 or 2 degrees are generated on the *mis*/kidding scale, the *mis*/kidding ranks as *mini*/kidding. See if you don't agree you've got better things to do with *your* time and energy than enforcing them:

Infancy

• Take as much formula for Daddy as you do for Mommy

• Don't cry when you see Grandma

• Stop throwing your pacifier on the floor

Toddlerhood

• Stop asking me to read a story after you've gone to bed

• Stop sucking your thumb

• Don't touch your (genitals – bellybutton, nose…..)

Preschooler

• Stop wetting the bed at night

• Eat your green vegetables

• Stop breath holding when you cry

Elementary Schooler

•Stop masturbating in your room

•Stop complaining about the clothes I select for you

•Make your bed as carefully as I do

Adolescence

- Don't waste your allowance on trash

- I don't care about the other kids, dress the way I tell you

- Do your homework as soon as you get home from school

Any of these examples, if persistent or intrusive enough, will eventually provoke more than a "cool" emotional reaction and will affect other Consequence Areas besides AUTHORITY. If the "heat" generated by persistence or intrusiveness of *mini*/kidding reaches 3 to 6 degrees, the *mini*/kidding becomes *Mid*/kidding and needs a plan for control. More about that in later chapters. Let's add what we've learned in this chapter to our developing strategy for managing *mis*/kidding.

Step Two toward Controlling *Mis*/kidding: Convert *KILLER*/kidding to *Mid*/kidding and Ignore *mini*/kidding

In real-life situations, *mis*/kidding kidding and good/*kidding* all occur together. Parents must identify *mis*/kidding and, after defining the *mis*/kidding with subjective and objective criteria, control any *KILLER*/kidding immediately. *Mini*/kidding is ignored until it goes away or until (because of its consequences on the kid or others) it becomes *Mid*/kidding. Success in controlling *mis*/kidding is achieved by converting all *mis*/kidding to *Mid*/kidding. This gives you time to find out reasons and plan a strategy. It ensures that your time and energy are not wasted.

Here are some examples of *mis*/kidding which include *KILLER*/kidding, *Mid*/kidding and *mini*/kidding. In each example of complex *mis*/kidding, *KILLER*/kidding is first converted to *Mid*/kidding and *mini*/kidding is ignored.

Converting *KILLER*/kidding To *Mid*/kidding In Two Preschoolers

Tommy and Bobby, aged 3 years, are playing near an open window in a third story apartment. Tommy suddenly stands and throws a metal matchbox car out the window and watches it smash on the ground. His friend Bobby climbs onto the windowsill to see more clearly. Mom turns and sees the boys.

Terrified, she grabs Bobby by the arm and yanks him to the floor. Bobby shrieks with freight, while Tommy screams, "Bad Mommy!" For several hours afterwards, Tommy refuses to hug his Mommy.

Discussion: Mommy recognizes Bobby on the windowsill as *KILLER*/kidding and stops it immediately. She ignores the boys' immediate reactions of crying and screaming at her as examples of *mini*/kidding. Tommy's refusal to hug her, another example of *mini*/kidding, is also ignored. If it were to persist, it would eventually become *Mid*/kidding and require management.

Converting *KILLER*/kidding To *Mid*/kidding In An Adolescent

Janet, 16 years of age, is seeing Hugh, 24 years old. She is failing her major subjects and her parents discover she has missed two weeks of school. Janet is caught selling marijuana at school. Court action is imminent. When her parents attempt to "ground" Janet to the home to stop her from seeing Hugh, she threatens to run away or take an overdose of pills. She claims that if her parents loved her, they would trust her more and let her see Hugh.

With the advice and support of their Pediatrician, the parents arrange for Janet's immediate admission to a "secure" adolescent psychiatric facility.

Discussion: Janet taking and selling drugs, as well as her threat to overdose on pills are *KILLER*/kidding. Her parents decide to stop the *KILLER*/kidding immediately by arranging a "secure" psychiatric hospital admission. The failing grades, playing hooky from school and the relationship with Hugh are *Mid*/kidding and require control, but there is time to develop a plan later. Janet's claims of not being loved and trusted are examples of *mini*/kidding and are ignored for the present. If they persist long enough to become *Mid*/kidding in their own right, time can be taken to deal with them.

If, in attempting to control the *KILLER*/kidding by hospitalizing Janet, she were to refuse to go to the hospital or attempt to run away, it would be appropriate to *forcefully restrain her and hospitalize her against her will.*

Now that you can identify *mis*/kidding (Chapter One) and categorize and convert it to *Mid*/kidding (Chapter Two), there is one more step to take before planning and carrying out a control strategy. You must decide how difficult it will be to manage and whether you'll need professional help to do it. The next chapter presents the things that make *mis*/kidding easy, difficult or impossible for you to control. You'll learn how to discover if kids are able to make better kidding choices or not, whether they're sick and how to use professional help.

In Summary:

To redirect *mis*/kidding-

- •Distinguish *KILLER*/kidding from *Mid*/kidding and mini/kidding

- •Convert *KILLER*/kidding to *Mid*/kidding with whatever force is needed

- •Ignore *mini*/kidding

1. Check your "subjective" emotional reaction to the *mis*/kidding and assign "degrees":

➤"HOT"   (FEAR)   = 3 degrees

➤"Warm" (Anxiety, Anger, Confusion)   = 2 degrees

➤"cool"   (annoyance)   = 1 degree

2. Check "objective" effects on Consequence Areas and count "degrees":

•AGE WORK..Up to 3 degrees

(*physical*)   =1

(*social*)   =1

(*communication*)   =1

•OTHERS...Up to 2 degrees

You   =1

Everyone else   =1

•AUTHORITY..1 degree

3. Add the "degrees" to define the *Mis*/kidding:

KILLER/kidding   =7 thru 9 degrees

Mid/kidding   =3, 4, 5, or 6 degrees

mini/kidding   =1 or 2 degrees

4. "Cool" *KILLER*/kidding to *Mid*/kidding immediately with whatever force is necessary and ignore *mini*/kidding.

CHAPTER THREE

IN/Kidding: The Mis/kidding That Needs Professionals

We've all watched a cat slink along a narrow fence and jump effortlessly to the ground. We've seen a male dog sniff and snort as it explores one garden spot or another, sometimes pausing to add its own contribution. These behaviors, alien to most humans, are easily recognized as typical of cats and dogs. We've seen kids shriek when separated from their mothers. We have no trouble (usually) telling cats, dogs and kids apart by their behaviors, though none of them may be house-trained! Even when we don't see an animal, but watch a talented mime or listen to a skilled storyteller, we can identify animals accurately. That's because each animal has its own pattern of behavior (and misbehavior). Each member of the group has enough similarities to each other member that its species can be recognized. These behaviors, caused by inheritance and physical make-up, are like the timbre of musical instruments. They're easy to recognize, whatever the activity, whatever the "tune."

Though we can recognize cats, dogs and kids by their innate behaviors, some cats learn to climb out of trees better than others, some dogs learn to hunt better than others, and some kids learn to separate from their mothers more easily than others. Within each species, environment (or experience) plays on inheritance (the body) to change behavior. Experience determines if a good/kidding "tune" will be played by the body. Just as what we hear from an instrument is the combined effect of its physical construction and the experience of the musician playing it, kidding is caused by the interplay of physical attributes and environmental experiences on kidding choices. Environmental experiences can be changed. By controlling or shaping them, kidding can be redirected. Physical endowment, like the construction of a musical instrument, is difficult or impossible to alter or rebuild without expert help.

In the last chapter you learned how to convert all *mis*/kidding to *Mid*/kidding. In this chapter we'll separate *Mid*/kidding due to "internal" causes, such as mental retardation, for which you may need professional help, from *Mid*/kidding due to "external" influences, which you can manage yourself.

"Internal" Causes of Mid/kidding: In/kidding

In/kidding is kidding caused by *events happening within kids, over which they have no control*. Because events happening within kids all find their roots within the skill areas of AGE WORK, In/kidding is expressed through *physical*, *social* and *communication* activities.

Normal physical and mental processes as well as injuries, whether obvious or hidden, insanity and other medical conditions are all manifested as In/kidding through their effects on AGE WORK. Other causes of In/kidding include congenital (from birth) and acquired mental and physical conditions. In/kidding can "warm up" to any degree of *mis*/kidding, from *mini*/kidding to *Mid*/kidding to *KILLER*/kidding. Since our strategy is to stop *KILLER*/kidding without taking time to discover causes, and to ignore *mini*/kidding, we need only examine *Mid*/kidding to see if it's caused by In/kidding. Soon I'll show you how to recognize In/kidding in any form it takes.

The importance of recognizing In/kidding when you encounter it is that you have only two choices to make to deal with it: (1) *Change what's happening inside the kid* and so change the In/kidding that's causing the *Mis*/kidding, or (2) *accept it and learn to live with it*.

Here are two examples of In/kidding where therapists or doctors can change what's happening in the kids:

> •Aborted suicide attempts due to depression - (Treated with psychotherapy, medicines).

> •Excessive soda drinking due to diabetes - (Treated with insulin).

Here are two examples of In/kidding that parents must learn to accept and live with:

> • "Immaturity" due to mental retardation - (Treated with special curriculum).

> • Inability to walk normally due to cerebral palsy - (Treated with physical and occupational therapy, braces, wheelchair).

Let's look a bit more closely at the alternatives of changing what's happening in kids versus learning to accept and live with limitations.

Controlling In/kidding By Changing What's Happening in Kids

Some causes of In/kidding, like depression and diabetes, can be controlled or corrected with accurate diagnosis and treatment. Without accurate diagnosis, neither condition is always recognized as a cause of *mis*/kidding. Attempted suicide might be ascribed to rebellion against authority without recognizing the underlying depression. Excessive thirst and weight loss might be interpreted as "diet mania" without recognition of the diabetes.

Depression and diabetes, lead poisoning and thyroid deficiency, and many other conditions, are among the potential "hidden causes" of In/kidding. When such conditions threaten or delay physical, social or communication skills, the components of AGE WORK, the delays can mistakenly be accepted as the "best the kids can do." Diagnosing the underlying conditions and changing what's happening in kids allows AGE WORK to progress, "cools" the *mis*/kidding and returns kidding choices to the kids.

Accepting In/kidding And Living with It

When In/kidding is truly caused by innate limitations in physical, social or communication skills, it's difficult or impossible to change. As we'll see in Chapters Four and Five, all our strategies to manage *Mid*/kidding depend on kids being free to make kidding choices. In/kidding, because it's not under kids' control, doesn't permit choice-making. When In/kidding can't be changed by changing what's happening in kids, parents can only accept and live with any *Mid*/kidding that results from it.

Cerebral palsy, mental retardation and autism, though treatable, are examples of conditions that impose innate limitations on AGE WORK. None of the treatments for these conditions, at least for now, can change the underlying causes for the resulting In/kidding. Once an accurate diagnosis is made, the focus of management is to help kids do their best with their limitations and for others to adjust their expectations to realistic levels.

Whenever you identify *Mid*/kidding that derives some of its "degrees" of "warmth" from AGE WORK, you need to know:

• Can you change what's happening in the kid to improve or protect the affected skill areas of AGE WORK and thus "cool" the *Mid*/kidding?

• Do you have to accept and live with the *Mid*/kidding because the affected skill areas of AGE WORK are innately deficient?

Before I acquaint you in detail with the professionals who help diagnose causes, let me show you how easy it is to recognize In/kidding. Recognizing In/kidding is your job. You don't need professionals to do it. In fact, as you'll see when we examine professionals more closely later in this chapter, some of them won't recognize In/kidding when it falls in another professional's field! Living with your kids makes *you* best at recognizing their In/kidding.

How to Recognize In/kidding

In recognizing In/kidding, understand that kids have *NO CHOICE* in acting it out. Diminished innate ability and internal processes like illness leave kids *NO CONTROL* over In/kidding. Internal processes and innate abilities all fall within the Consequence Area of AGE WORK, so the first test for In/kidding is to see whether it generates at least 1 "degree" of its "warmth" on the *mis*/kidding scale from AGE WORK. *Mis*/kidding with normal AGE WORK can't be In/kidding (though we'll see what it is, later in this chapter). If AGE WORK is involved in defining the *mis*/kidding, it may be In/kidding and you'll need a second test. Use Appendix I to identify delays in AGE WORK.

The second and most reliable test for In/kidding is to check its "look" and "feel." *Mid*/kidding done without choice or control looks and feels very different from that done with choice and control. You already know what observing *Mid*/kidding feels like; Confusion, Anxiety or Anger, the subjective criteria of *Mid*/kidding. To pin down In/kidding most reliably as the cause of *Mid*/kidding, observe both what it feels like *and* what it looks like. Here's how it's done:

In/kidding- Its Look And Feel

What It Looks Like	*What It Feels Like*
(Your Observation)	(Your Emotional Reaction)

The Mid/kidding doesn't make sense

•It happens unpredictably   Confusion

•It targets everyone (non-selective)

....AND/OR...............................

•There's <u>no benefit</u> to the kid

•It <u>threatens or hurts</u> the kid   Anxiety

(I'll be talking about Anger as a reaction to *Mid*/kidding and what causes it later on in this chapter).

Many hidden causes are possible and some are listed, but you don't need to know any of them to <u>recognize</u> the *Mid*/kidding as In/kidding. Use Appendix I to identify delays in Age Work, a reliable indicator of In/kidding. Here follow some examples of the *look* and *feel* of In/kidding:

<u>In an infant</u>: Normal eight-month-old babies can sleep through the night most of the time without feedings. They can sit without support and coo at their parents. An infant who fails to achieve these milestones shows delays in AGE WORK.

Mid/kidding	AGE WORK Delayed *skill area*	Possible In/kidding	It's *In*/kidding When: The "*Look*" The "*Feel*"
Baby never sits	*Physical*	Muscle disease Brain damage	**Non-selective** *Anxiety* **No benefit**
Won't stop crying	*Physical Social*	Pain No bonding	**Non-selective** *Anxiety* **No benefit**
Coos at no one	*Social Communication*	No bonding Deafness	**Non-selective** *Anxiety* **No benefit**

If this baby shrieked and refused to sit or coo whenever the grandparents held it, but calmed itself and sat and cooed for its parents, the *mis*/kidding wouldn't be "random" or "non-selective." It could be "beneficial" to the baby and would make sense if the baby wanted to be with its parents. None of the adults, observing this, would feel Anxiety or Confusion, though the grandparents might feel annoyance or even Anger. The *mis*/kidding wouldn't qualify as In/kidding.

Here are two other examples of the *look* and *feel* of In/kidding. As before, you don't need to know the causes to *recognize* the In/kidding, though some possible internal causes are shown:

<u>In an elementary schooler</u>: Elementary schoolers can hold pencils to write. They attend to their bathroom needs and talk to their teachers. An elementary schooler who can't hold a pencil, wets or soils clothing, or doesn't speak intelligibly demonstrates delays in AGE WORK.

Mid/kidding	AGE WORK Delayed *skill area*	Possible In/kidding	It's *In*/kidding When: The *"Look"* The *"Feel"*
Can't hold a pencil	*Physical*	Cerebral palsy Myasthenia gravis	Non-selective *Anxiety* No benefit
Wets and soils	*Physical Social*	Spinal tumor Autism	Non-selective *Anxiety* No benefit
Speech unintelli-gible	*Physical Communication*	Cleft palate Mental retardation	Non-selective *Confusion* No benefit

In An Adolescent: Adolescents should be able to engage in physical education activities at school. They're expected to maintain friendships without the help of drunk driving and to maintain passing grades. When a teenager's stamina and coordination deteriorate, friendships dry up, leading to isolation, and grades suddenly fall, AGE WORK is threatened.

Mid/kidding	AGE WORK Delayed *skill area*	Possible In/kidding	It's *In*/kidding When: The *"Look"* The *"Feel"*
Poor stamina, coordination	*Physical*	Drug abuse Muscular dystrophy	Non-selective *Anxiety* Threatening
Losing friends	*Social*	Tourette Syndrome Depression	No benefit *Anxiety*
Failing grades	*Communication*	ADHD Alcoholism	No benefit *Confusion* Threatening *Anxiety*

Internal, (often hidden) processes, at work at all times and in all places, cause In/kidding *without obvious reason*. When In/kidding reaches the *Mid*/kidding level, it causes the *Mid*/kidding to be *unpredictable, non-selective* of its target, of no benefit to kids and often *threatening*. When you look at *Mid*/kidding that affects AGE WORK, doesn't make sense, and makes you feel Confused or Anxious, assume it's In/kidding. Before you can control or manage In/kidding at the *Mid*/kidding level, you must discover how much it limits kids' abilities to make choices. You need to find out whether, by treating its causes, you can unmask "normal" skills that would allow better kidding choices, or if the *Mid*/kidding reflects innate limitations you'll have to live with.

Now that you can recognize In/kidding, let's see how its causes can be diagnosed:

In/kidding: The Mid/kidding That Needs Professionals

No matter how expert we are, even if we're child specialists, neither you nor I will ever be able to recognize all the "hidden causes" of In/kidding without help. That's because some hidden causes masquerade as others and require special tests or techniques to be diagnosed. For example, lead poisoning can masquerade as mental retardation or a learning disability. Thyroid deficiency, depression and many other conditions can do the same. Once we've identified In/kidding at the *Mid*/kidding level, we need an accurate diagnosis of the cause. That's the only way we can discover what kids' true abilities are and how much choice they have over the *Mid*/kidding.

Over the years, I've narrowed the field of professional In/kidding helpers down to three major categories: Physicians, Psychologists and Educators.

There's an easy way to choose the right kind of professional(s) to diagnose causes of In/kidding:

• When Physical skills are impaired, choose a Physician

• When Social skills are compromised, choose a Psychologist

• When Communication skills are lagging, choose an Educator

Here's a diagram illustrating what you've learned about *Mid*/kidding due to In/kidding and its relationship to AGE WORK and the other Consequence Areas:

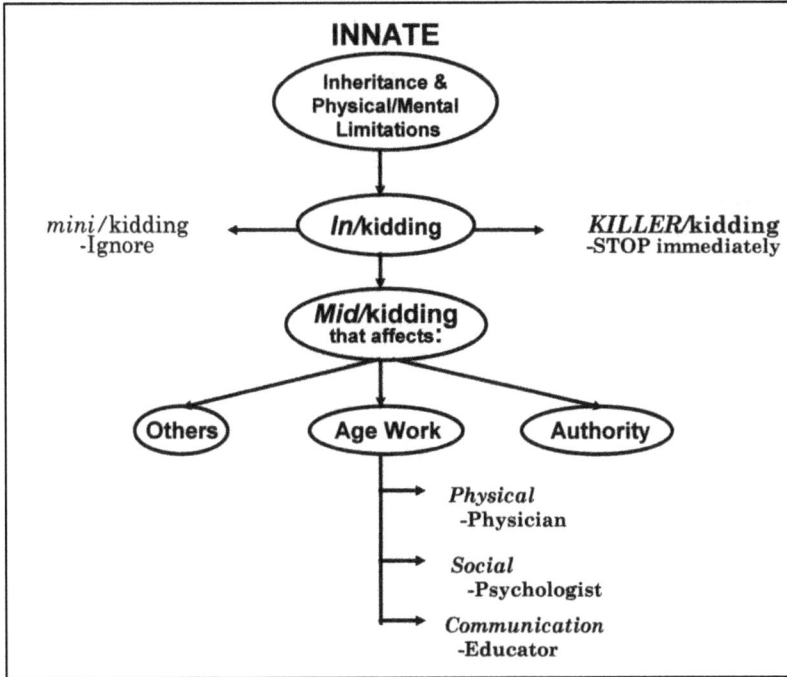

When two or more areas of AGE WORK are affected by *Mid*/kidding, I suggest choosing professionals in the following order: Physician (physical) Psychologist (social) Educator (communication). If several professionals are needed, because several areas of AGE WORK are involved, consulting professionals in this order will give you the best chance for proper diagnosis and treatment of the problem. In general, physical problems must be controlled before social problems can be solved and social problems must be solved before communication problems can be remediated.

In/kidding doesn't always require a professional for diagnosis or control. A two year old repeatedly reaching for icing on a birthday cake in the kitchen is In/kidding. This toddler's social skills haven't matured enough to allow him to be left alone with the cake. Recognizing this, you'll likely feel, annoyance registering only 1 "cool" subjective "degree." You may consider your AUTHORITY threatened, generating 1 more "cool" objective degree. You won't need a professional with this type of *mini*/kidding to tell you to separate the kid from the cake! But if a two year old has a bizarre appetite and eats dirt, raids garbage cans and craves drinking toilet water, you'll likely feel Confusion or Anxiety, yielding 2 "warm" subjective degrees. The possibility of this *mis*/kidding causing infection or poisoning within the physical area of AGE WORK creates another degree, totaling at least 3 "degrees" on the *mis*/kidding scale. In/kidding that "warms up" to the *Mid*/kidding level does require professional help; in this example, from a Physician and a Psychologist.

Tell Me Again; How Do I Decide I Need Professional Help?

Chapter One: Recognize *mis*/kidding by seeing if the kidding affects any of the Consequence Areas of AGE WORK, OTHERS or AUTHORITY.

Chapter Two: Redirect the *mis*/kidding by converting any *KILLER*/Kidding to *Mid*/kidding, with overwhelming force, if needed, and ignore *mini*/kidding.

Chapter Three: Recognize In/kidding by its effects on AGE WORK and by its "look" (unpredictable, non-selective, no benefit, threatening) and "feel" (Anxiety or Confusion). Consult with a professional for each affected skill area of AGE WORK, in the following order:

• Physical: choose a Physician

• Social: choose a Psychologist

• Communication: choose an Educator

Now that you know if you need professional help and what categories of professionals are best equipped to diagnose and manage In/kidding, you need to learn a little about the qualifications of the specialists in each discipline.

Though there are more names for specialists that work with *mis*/kidding than there are pages in this book, they all fall into one or another of the categories of Physicians, Psychologists, or Educators. Each group, like cats, dogs and kids, have certain "innate differences", making it easy to tell one "species" from another. And like cats, dogs and kids, different experts within each category have learned to solve certain kinds of *mis*/kidding problems better than others. In the pages that follow, the capabilities of each professional discipline and some of the peculiarities of its members are presented.

Physicians and In/kidding

Physicians are medical doctors who are licensed to treat people with prescription medicines, hospitalization and/or surgery. Pediatricians are physicians who treat kids - often through twenty years of age. They may further specialize and treat intellectual or neurological deficits (Developmental Pediatricians), behavioral or learning problems (Behavioral Pediatricians), brain and nervous system conditions (Pediatric Neurologists), or severe emotional states (Child Psychiatrists).

All physicians use similar steps to help solve a problem. First, they take a history. This means they ask lots of questions about how kids got to be the way they are. Always included are questions about physical growth and development as well as possible diseases that may have contributed to the problem. Next, they perform a physical examination. Child Psychiatrists, to avoid frightening a kid, will often ask a pediatrician or other physician to do the physical examination to be sure no disease is present. Last, a treatment is recommended, often in the form of a prescription.

Physicians are trained to look for causes. When you suspect physical problems are causing delays in AGE WORK, physicians can help you find out "why." As you've seen, finding causes is essential to deciding if In/kidding can be changed by treatment or if you have to accept the *mis*/kidding and live with it.

• General and Family Practitioners, Internists and Pediatricians are all "generalists" who can sort out problems. Any one of them may know you and your family well enough to recognize *mis*/kidding, but may not have specialized training to solve the problem. In such cases, these physicians may refer you to other physician-specialists who can solve the problem.

• Developmental/Behavioral Pediatricians have studied normal brain development in kids. They have learned psychiatric and psychological techniques to identify *mis*/kidding problems, especially *physical*ly-based In/kidding. Though they are trained to assess the *social* and *communication* components of AGE WORK as well, they do not usually treat these problems independently. For psychotherapy or remediation of educational disorders, these physicians usually refer to psychologists or educators.

• Child Neurologists specialize in *physical* disorders of the brain and nervous system. When *mis*/kidding is suspected to be caused by a physical condition that seems to be getting worse, or in which ongoing damage to the nervous system may be occurring, Child Neurologists can perform necessary tests to diagnose and organize treatment for the condition. These physicians are not "generalists" and should not be asked to "sort out" causes for *mis*/kidding.

• Child Psychiatrists have training in child neurology, but do not usually do a physical examination. It is to the Child Psychiatrist that a kid is referred after physical disease has been ruled out. Often, another professional will have diagnosed a problem in the social component of AGE WORK (e.g. "emotional disturbance") that requires either a medicine or a search for a non-physical cause of the *mis*/kidding. Child Psychiatrists can be very costly, but while they are providing therapy, they, like other physicians, are able to prescribe medicines or hospitalize kids. Like Child Neurologists, Child Psychiatrists are not "generalists" and should not be asked to "sort out" *mis*/kidding problems.

Psychologists and In/kidding

Psychologists can be described as "those who study the workings of the mind; especially feelings, desires and mental processes." By this definition, there are many more kinds of "psychologists" than there are types of physicians. If we limit ourselves to those "psychologists" who study and treat humans, and especially kids, it will be easier to understand this "species." Even so, you need to know that some "psychologists" are called Social Workers, while some professionals called "School Psychologists" are really Educators (we'll learn about them below).

Psychologists who diagnose and treat kids are certified or licensed to do so. They are not medical doctors, though they may have either a Ph.D. (Doctor of Philosophy in Psychology), a Psy.D. (Doctor of Psychology), an M.A. or M.S. (Master of Arts or Science), or other advanced degree. They do not perform physical examinations on kids, but rather assess problems by using tests of intelligence, achievement, educational skills or emotional functioning. All members of this "species" give therapy, but the range of services differs for each one. In the following paragraphs I'll describe some of the differences that are important in helping you decide which to use. Some individual psychologists do not follow the general statements made here. I strongly suggest you check with any psychologist you plan to use before committing to that individual to be sure the service you need is provided. For example, if people at different stages of life are having difficulty in your family, choose a psychologist who specializes in family therapy.

• Clinical Child Psychologists are doctoral level experts who assess and give therapy for *mis*/kidding affecting the *social* component of AGE WORK. Though they also diagnose *mis*/kidding affecting the *communication* component of AGE WORK, after diagnosis, such problems are referred for remediation to Educators, a third group of professionals discussed below. There are two subcategories within the group of Clinical Child Psychologists; Analytic and Behavioral Psychologists:

• Analytic Child Psychologists follow the psychiatric tradition and spend considerable time searching for causes of *mis*/kidding. Sometimes years are spent in analysis, looking for causes in what a kid says and does. The goal is to help develop "insight" or understanding, and so help the kid control or change the *mis*/kidding.

• Behavioral Child Psychologists focus on the actual behavior. After collecting information about the *mis*/kidding, a plan or strategy is designed to change it. This is more direct than the analytic approach, and I recommend it because it's faster and less costly. If it fails to work after an adequate trial, you can always reconsider the insight approach.

•Psychiatric Social Workers are a special group of Social Workers who diagnose and give therapy for *mis*/kidding affecting the *social* component of AGE WORK. They can also assess *mis*/kidding affecting the *communication* component of AGE WORK, but refer such problems to Educators for remediation. Psychiatric Social Workers usually have a master's degree, though some have a doctorate. Social Workers' additional knowledge about society's systems and agencies may be of particular benefit in cases, for example, of juvenile delinquency, drug, sex or physical abuse.

When you identify *mis*/kidding affecting the *social* skill area of AGE WORK, and it causes Anxiety or Confusion, a Psychologist is the best type of professional to start with. If the psychologist suspects In/kidding affecting the *physical* or *communication* skill areas of AGE WORK, referral will be made to a Physician or an Educator.

Let's look at the third category of professionals, the Educators. Within this group are School Psychologists. Those School Psychologists who are found exclusively within schools and do not give therapy, I classify as Educators rather than Psychologists.

Educators and In/kidding

A common element in the category of Educators is that they focus on the education of kids in schools, whether day by day classroom instruction, assessment and remediation of academic performance, or administration of the school and its staff. These professionals do not perform physical examinations, write medical prescriptions or give psychotherapy. Though Educators assess school-related problems using a variety of tests, they rarely search for basic causes. Their evaluations help to define *mis*/kidding and label it. This information is then used to develop an Individual Educational Program, or IEP, to assist the kid in learning.

Educators comprise the most diverse of the categories of professionals. They include:

•Principals (and Vice Principals)

•Teachers

•School Counselors; Pupil Personnel Workers

•School Psychologists (Educational Psychologists, Psychometrists)

•Educational Specialists (math, speech and language, reading)

•Occupational and Physical Therapists (Perceptual-Motor Specialists)

•Audiologists

•School Nurses

When you identify In/kidding affecting the communication skill area of AGE WORK, and it causes Anxiety or Confusion, an Educator is the best professional to begin with. If the Educator suspects In/kidding due to a physical or social component of AGE WORK, referral will be made to a Physician or a Psychologist.

One last word about *mis*/kidding and professionals. Sometimes, you won't know how to convert *KILLER*/kidding to *Mid*/kidding without help.

Whenever you encounter *KILLER*/kidding you need to STOP, look at the skill areas of AGE WORK if affects. Use those skill areas to choose a professional helper in this order:

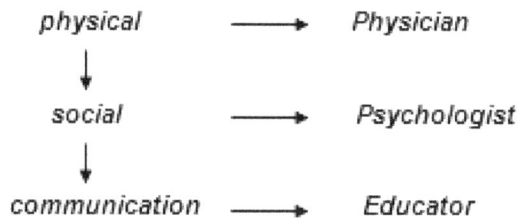

physical   ⟶   Physician

↓

social   ⟶   Psychologist

↓

communication   ⟶   Educator

For more advice on choosing the right expert within each category of professionals and how you stay in charge of making decisions about the *Mis*/kidding while you get the help, read More About Professionals in **Appendix Two**. There, you also learn how to talk to professionals, how to limit what they do and when to fire them.

This is a good place for you to stop a moment and take a bow! You began your venture in *MIS*/KIDDING by observing with me an infinite variety of kidding. You've then recognized and separated *mis*/kidding from all the other kidding activities. Next, you've forcefully eliminated *KILLER*/kidding, turned away from *mini*/kidding, and limited your focus to *Mid*/kidding. Finally, by isolating In/kidding, for which you may need professional help, you've learned how much of the *Mid*/kidding you'll have to live with.

Now there remains only the type of *Mid*/kidding that kids engage in by choice and which either annoys you or makes you Angry when you observe it. Having removed all other forms of *mis*/kidding from your immediate attention, you've given yourself time to develop strategies for its control. This residual *Mid*/kidding, sparked by events occurring "outside" kids' bodies, and to which they choose their responses, I call Out/kidding. It's the focus of the remaining chapters of this book.

"External" Causes Of Mid/kidding: Out/kidding

Out/kidding is kidding provoked by events occurring outside a kid. When Out/kidding "warms up" to *mis*/kidding at the *Mid*/kidding level, it needs to be controlled because it harms kids or others over time. Since experiences, or the effects of environment, determine Out/kidding, it can be controlled by altering kids' experiences. Instead of allowing experiences to occur randomly, you can devise them to curb or shape Out/kidding.

Besides experiences that you can control, "environment" includes kids' interactions with other people and other things which you may not be able to control. Television and movies, family and community, even climate, cause Out/kidding. To manage Out/kidding at the *Mid*/kidding level, the experiences you control must be made more meaningful (or more powerful) than those you cannot control. In Chapter Five I'll show you how to make experiences you control more compelling than others in the environment.

Here's a diagram that shows the relationship between Out/kidding, the environment, and you:

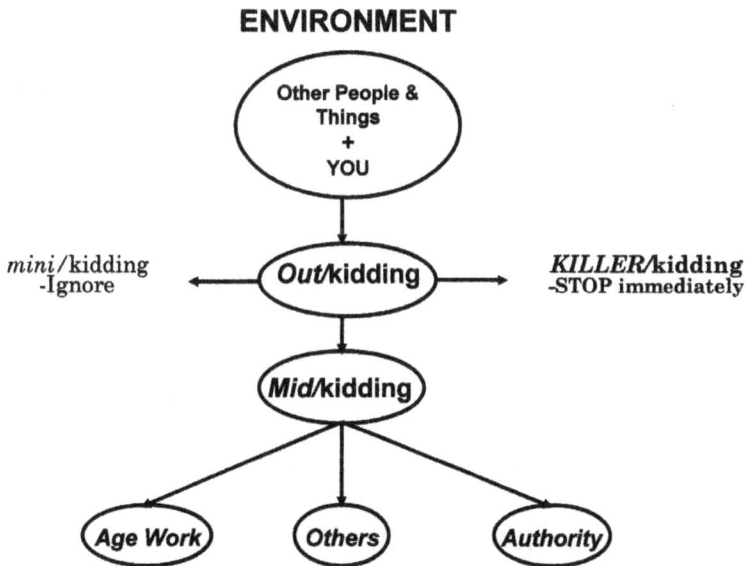

ENVIRONMENT

Other People &
Things
+
YOU

mini/kidding
-Ignore   ← Out/kidding →   *KILLER*/kidding
-STOP immediately

Mid/kidding

Age Work   Others   Authority

Just as you can recognize In/kidding by its "look" and "feel" without relying on professionals, you can recognize Out/kidding by its own "look" and "feel."

How To Recognize Out/kidding

The key to recognizing Out/kidding is to understand that kids engage in it *by choice*. Because they choose Out/kidding, kids decide when it happens, to whom it's directed and what they hope to achieve by it. Since this *Mid*/kidding is contrived, though not always consciously, it may target only one or another selected Consequence Area. Unlike In/kidding, Out/kidding doesn't always involve AGE WORK, but it does always affect someone's AUTHORITY. The challenge to AUTHORITY, so typical of Out/kidding, leads the observer away from the feeling of Anxiety or Confusion evoked by In/kidding, and ignites feelings of annoyance or Anger:

Out/kidding- Its Look And Feel

What It *Looks* Like (Your Observation)	What It *Feels* Like (Your Emotional Reaction)
The *Mid*/kidding *is manipulative.*	
• It's <u>predictable</u>.	*annoyance*
• It's <u>selective</u>; some people, not others.	
....**AND/OR**...	
• It <u>challenges</u> someone's AUTHORITY, forcing them to do or allow something unacceptable.	*Anger*

When Out/kidding challenges AUTHORITY and seems to indicate kids are doing whatever they want, you can be sure their actions were chosen for a reason and the reason is always the same. Kids choose Out/kidding because they anticipate desirable (from their perspective, naturally) consequences. This is the essence of Out/kidding: The environment within which kids devise their actions to achieve (what they consider) desirable consequences, is accessible at only certain times and at certain places. The former attribute makes Out/kidding predictable, while the latter makes it selective. The predictable and selective challenge to AUTHORITY, characteristic of Out/kidding, is what provokes subjective feelings of annoyance or Anger in the observer.

Here's an example of the look and feel of Out/kidding. You'll notice some similarities between it and an example of In/kidding you examined earlier. You'll see that Out/kidding always affects AUTHORITY, while it may or may not affect AGE WORK and OTHERS. Note that rather than provoking feelings of Confusion or Anxiety, Out/kidding at the *Mid*/kidding level kindles annoyance or Anger in the observer. Though kids engage in Out/kidding to achieve their own ends, you don't need to know what's motivating them for you to recognize the Out/kidding. Here are some examples:

In an infant: Grandparents report that an eight month old infant arches its back, shrieks and never coos at them when it's held on their laps. Later, with the parents, the baby sits calmly and coos. If the grandparents see a threat to their AUTHORITY (1 degree), a threat to the social skill area of AGE WORK (1 degree), an ill-effect on their relationship to the baby as a pair of OTHERS (1 degree), and feel annoyed (1 degree), they've defined *Mid*/kidding. Though the *Mid*/kidding affects AGE WORK, it must be Out/kidding because it's predictable, selective and challenges their AUTHORITY.

Out/kidding	Consequence Areas	Possible Cause For Out/kidding	It's Out/kidding When: The "Look" The "Feel"
Baby shrieks; won't sit or coo.	AUTHORITY (1°) OTHERS (1°) AGE WORK -*social* (1°)	Fright Wants parents	Selective *annoyance* Predictable (1°) Total: 4 degrees

(*Mid*/kidding = 3-6 degrees)

Sometimes, you'll tally up enough *mis*/kidding "degrees" to define *Mid*/kidding, but you'll feel both annoyance (or Anger) and Confusion (or Anxiety); that is, the subjective criteria for both Out/kidding and In/kidding. Don't panic! Trust your feelings; both kinds of *Mid*/kidding are present and you'll need professional help to diagnose causes for the In/kidding before you do anything with the Out/kidding. Identify the skill areas of AGE WORK that are causing the confusion or anxiety to get the proper expert help. In real-life, kids have "as many diseases as they pleases!" Here's an example:

In an elementary schooler: A math teacher reports that an elementary schooler keeps calling out and dropping his pencil in class. Lessons are disrupted when classmates laugh and become unruly. Neither his parents nor other teachers see this occur elsewhere.

Since the math teacher's AUTHORITY (1 degree) is threatened, OTHERS, including the teacher, are disturbed (2 degrees), and the math teacher is annoyed (1 degree), *Mid*/kidding is defined:

Out/kidding	Consequence Areas	Possible Cause For Out/kidding	It's Out/kidding When: The "Look" The "Feel"
Calls out, drops pencil when in math class	AUTHORITY (1°) OTHERS (2°) -Others (1°) -You (1°)	"Class clown" or Unprepared	Selective & *annoyance* Predictable (1°) Total: 4 degrees

(*Mid*/kidding = 3-6 degrees)

Because this *Mid*/kidding is predictable and selective (it occurs only in math class), challenges AUTHORITY and provokes annoyance, it must be Out/kidding.

Now imagine the same scenario with one difference; all the teachers (and the parents) notice the student's fingers getting weaker and weaker over several weeks until he no longer can hold a pencil. The effects of this *mis*/kidding may still annoy the math teacher, but Confusion or Anxiety will also be provoked. Dropping pencils everywhere with progressive weakness of the fingers is non-selective, of no benefit, Anxiety-provoking (or Confusing), and affects the physical skill area of AGE WORK. This qualifies as In/kidding and will require diagnosis by a physician before a strategy can be developed for the *Mid*/kidding:

Mid/kidding	Consequence Areas	Possible In/kidding	It's In/kidding When: The "Look" The "Feel"
Progressive weakness, drop pencils everywhere	OTHERS (2°) -Others (1°) -You (1°) AGE WORK (1°) -physical	Myasthenia Muscular dystrophy Lead poisoning	Non-selective & *Anxiety* (2°) No benefit Total: 5 degrees

Calling out only in math class, still predictable, selective and annoying, remains an example of Out/kidding.

How To Simplify Complex Mis/kidding

Complex *mis*/kidding, representing all the "bad stuff" kids do, is nothing more than In/kidding, Out/kidding or a mixture of both, reaching levels of *mini*/kidding, *Mid*/kidding or *KILLER*/kidding.

Once you've isolated *Mid*/kidding by stopping the *KILLER*/kidding and ignoring the *mini*/kidding, separate In/kidding from Out/kidding by using the criteria you've just learned. Remember, In/kidding is non-selective, unpredictable, of no benefit to kids and often threatening. It will Confuse you or make you feel Anxious and will always affect one or more skill area of AGE WORK. For each skill area affected there is a professional discipline to help diagnose the cause; Physicians for *physical* skills, Psychologists for *social* skills, and Educators for *communication* skills. Learn if you can change the In/kidding, or whether you have to accept it and live with it, by getting help from one, two or all three professional disciplines before you attempt to manage the residual Out/kidding.

What's So Important about Limiting Mis/kidding To Out/kidding?

All your efforts thus far have been directed toward identifying, sorting out and reducing complex *mis*/kidding to Out/kidding at the *Mid*/kidding level. This diagnostic phase of the *MIS*/KIDDING process ensures that the simple, but powerful, techniques you learn in the management phase, presented next, will be effective. Since kids engage in Out/kidding as a matter of choice, and always with the anticipation of desirable consequences, controlling Out/kidding becomes a matter of deciding on good/kidding commands, then energizing the commands by offering kids consequences they can't refuse. The management phase of the *MIS*/KIDDING process is the subject of Part Two of this book.

In Summary:

Isolate In/*kidding by-*

1. Identifying *Mid/*kidding that affects AGE WORK and-

"*looks*" -	and	"*feels*"-
• *non-selective*		**Confusing**
• *unpredictable*		or
• *of no benefit*		**Anxiety**-provoking

Choosing a professional for each affected *skill area* of AGE WORK,

in this order:

physical   ⟶   **PHYSICIAN**

↓

social   ⟶   **PSYCHOLOGIST**

↓

communication   ⟶   **EDUCATOR**

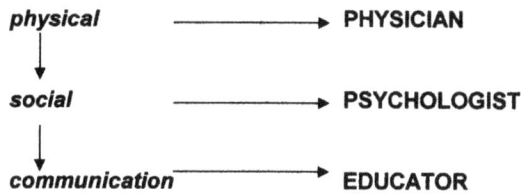

Be certain only Out/*kidding remains by-*

Checking to see that the *Mid/*kidding-

"*looks*"-	an	"*feels*"-
• *selective*		**annoying**
• *predictable*		or
• *challenging to AUTHORITY*		**Anger**-provoking

Part Two

Defining Good/kidding: Word Language Commands

The next three chapters present the management phase of the *MIS*/KIDDING process.

Here's where you learn to:

- Decide what you want your kid to do instead of *mis*/kidding.

- Get your kid to do it.

- Use the *MIS*/KIDDING process for even the most complex *mis*/kidding problems.

CHAPTER FOUR

Defining Good/kidding: Word Language Commands

You've just seen how Out/kidding at the *Mid*/kidding level provokes annoyance or Anger by assaulting AUTHORITY. You've learned that kids always have reasons for Out/kidding and the reasons are always the same; anticipation of desirable consequences from their viewpoint. When kids choose to do something they're not supposed to do or refuse to do something they should do, they perceive the anticipated consequences of their activity (or inactivity) to be more seductive or compelling than any other consequences within their environment.

We'll explore environmental experiences and how they affect kidding choices in a moment, but first, let's categorize the Out/kidding choices kids make.

The "Energy Content" Of Out/kidding: Active and Passive Out/kidding

Choosing to do things they're not supposed to do, when it's at the *Mid*/kidding level, is an active form of *mis*/kidding that demands energy from kids. The greater the number of "degrees" on the *mis*/kidding thermometer, the greater the amount of energy required. When you devise a strategy to control active *Mid*/kidding, you'll do best if you utilize that *mis*guided energy to promote good/kidding rather than trying to obliterate and squander it.

Of course, if you're a baby-sitter or other part-time person in authority and have only limited time to react to *Mid*/kidding, obliterating it may be all you have time to do. For a full-time authority person, like a parent or grandparent, harnessing the energy of active Out/kidding, especially when it's intense, gives you an opportunity to move kids furthest along the path toward adulthood.

Here are some examples of active Out/kidding at the *Mid*/kidding level:

•A ten month old baby crying whenever its parents put it down

• A three year old hitting its playmates, unprovoked

• A ten year old using foul language in school

• A sixteen year old taking parents' belongings without permission

When kids refuse to do things they're supposed to do, and their *mis*/kidding "warms up" to the *Mid*/kidding level, they're engaging in passive Out/kidding. The energy kids devote to passive Out/kidding is much less than that for active Out/kidding, so there's less *mis*guided energy to harness. As a result, your strategy for managing passive Out/kidding will be to create motivation for kids to pursue good/kidding goals.

Here are some examples of passive Out/kidding at the *Mid*/kidding level:

• A ten month old refusing to hold its bottle

• A three year old communicating only by gesture to a certain teacher

• A ten year old failing to turn off the TV when finished

• A sixteen year old consistently leaving dirty clothes on the bedroom floor

Remember, whenever kids fail to do what they're supposed to do, you need to test for the presence of In/kidding. You need to be sure kids are *refusing* to perform rather than being *unable* to perform. If In/kidding is suspected, diagnose the causes and find out if you can change them or if you have to accept and live with them. If necessary, consult the appropriate professional(s) before going any further. You can manage active or passive Out/kidding at the *Mid*/kidding level with the techniques you're about to learn, but In/kidding at any level takes away kids' choice-making and must be recognized and excluded before proceeding.

Now it's time to explore the experiences that lure kids toward Out/kidding and the environment within which you can influence their kidding choices. Recall for a moment our diagram of environmental influences affecting Out/kidding:

The environmental "bubble" at the top of the diagram (next page) includes OTHER PEOPLE and THINGS and YOU. These components of kids' surroundings create the experiences that tempt kids to engage in Out/kidding. Though kidsexperience their environment through all the five senses of hearing, vision, taste,touch and smell, by far the two most influential experiences are what kids hear and what they see. Kids are always listening and watching how OTHERPEOPLE and THINGS and YOU react to their kidding. Since you may not have control over what OTHER PEOPLE and THINGS communicate to kids, YOU, as an authority person, must become the vehicle for managing their Out/kidding.

ENVIRONMENT

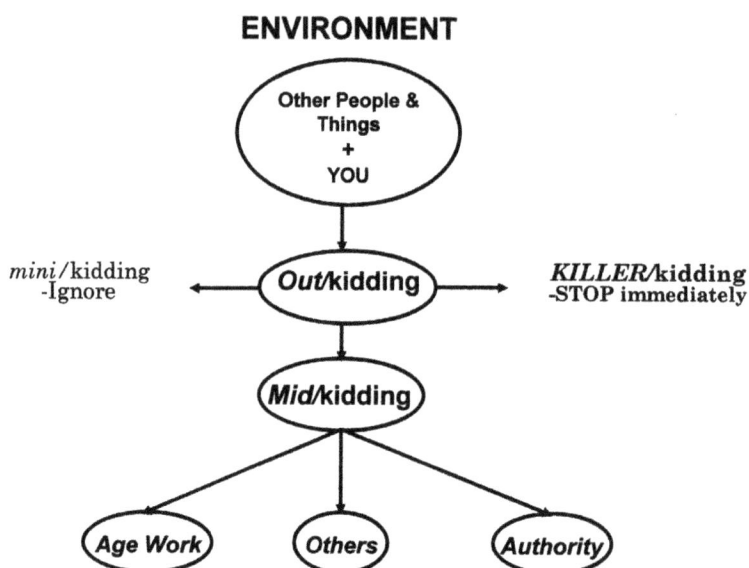

Communication from the Environment: Word Language vs. Action Language

Environmental experiences are created by what you are saying as well as your actions and those of other people and things in the vicinity of kids. What the environment "says" and what it "does" comprise forms of language. I call what kids hear, Word Language (W/L), and what they see (and feel, taste and smell), Action Language (A/L).

If you tell kids what they're doing is "good," you communicate Word Language (W/L). If, while doing what they're doing, kids experience something pleasant (see, feel, taste or smell), that's Action Language (A/L). Likewise, if you tell kids what they're doing is "bad", undesirable or dangerous, you communicate W/L, but when kids experience something unpleasant or painful as a result of their actions, that's A/L.

If you act differently from the way you say you do, kids believe what they see rather than what they hear. That's because A/L is inherently more "honest" than W/L due to its greater consistency. If you, as a part of the environment, tell kids through W/L that their *Mid*/kidding is undesirable or unacceptable, kids check the surrounding A/L (including yours) for consistency, their test for "honesty." When W/L is inconsistent with A/L (or "dishonest"), kids act in accordance with A/L.

Let's look at the outline of a powerful motor you can create for kid control.

It's "wired" with W/L and "activated" with A/L, and it can control active or passive *Mid*/kidding.

W/L Commands & A/L Consequences: The "Motor" For Kid Control

W/L (what you say) expresses your wishes. Even when wishes are voiced as commands, they're only wishes and have no power of their own. W/L is like the wiring of a motor; someone's physical design to guide energy through a device to activate it. I call W/L designed to control Out/kidding, Word Language Commands (W/L Commands). I've chosen the term "Commands" rather than "suggestions" or "choices" because, having passed through the steps of defining Out/kidding, we won't be negotiating with kids about the need for managing the *mis*/kidding, but only about the options within the commands they may choose.

A/L (things kids experience) in the vicinity of YOU, OTHER PEOPLE and THINGS is like formless energy; it crackles and pops in all directions, sometimes pleasant, sometimes hurtful. When A/L is directed to follow W/L Commands, it "activates" the motor for kid control. I call A/L contrived to activate W/L Commands, Action Language Consequences.

The components of every "motor" used for kid control in *MIS*/KIDDING will always be the same; a W/L Command, connected to an A/L Consequence. The design of each "motor" will vary with its function. Motors used for active Out/kidding are designed differently than those used for passive Out/kidding.

Those used by (full-time) parents are of a different power than those used by part-time authority persons, like babysitters.

In the remainder of this chapter, I'll show you how to choose W/L Commands for different types of Out/kidding and for the different roles you may assume as a caretaker of kids. In Chapter Five, I'll teach you how to "activate" your commands by using powerful A/L Consequences.

"Wiring" W/L Commands for Active Out/kidding - Managing Misdirected Energy: Deterrence, Deflection or Diversion

There are only three types of W/L Commands that control active Out/kidding.

When kids choose to do things they're not supposed to do, you can *deter*, *deflect* or *divert* their *mis*/kidding. The "wiring" diagram for each of these types of kid control "motors" is a bit different and each requires a bit different strategy by the authority person. Depending upon the time and energy you have in your authority role, you may find one or another of these W/L Commands most suitable.

To better understand the strengths and weaknesses of Deterrence, Deflection and Diversion, let's diagram what's happening with kids who are actively Out/kidding. The process is always the same; kids are actively pursuing an inappropriate goal that they find desirable:

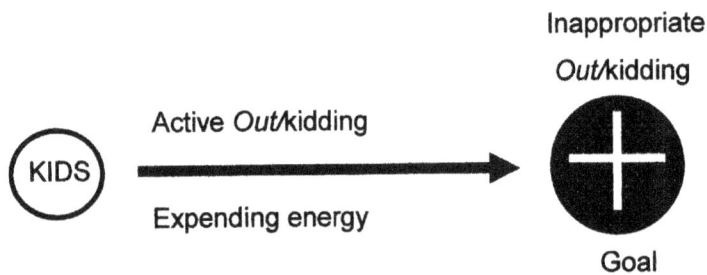

In active Out/kidding, shown above, kids expend energy trying to reach a (misdirected) Out/kidding goal. Rather than being apathetic or inert, kids are actually motivated, often highly motivated, to achieve an inappropriate goal.

Blocking or Deterring Out/kidding with a barrier at least as powerful as kids' misdirected motivation is the fastest, but most energy-wasting, of the W/LCommands. If you, as an authority person, stand directly in the path of kids'active Out/kidding efforts, you'll need to expend at least as much energy as the kids do to block them. Since W/L is merely a wish without an A/L Consequence, the W/L Command must be "activated" with an A/L Consequence. W/L Commands in the Deterrence mode are diagrammed below:

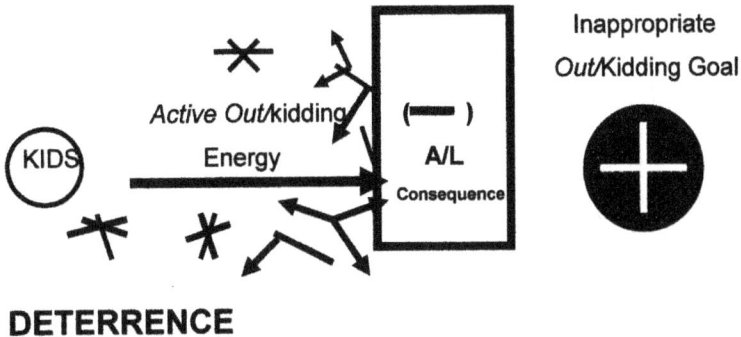

DETERRENCE

Note that the deterrent to kids achieving their Out/kidding goal is an unpleasant (-) A/L Consequence. See how kids' misdirected energies "splatter" against the (-) barrier. Those energies are wasted since they're not redirected toward good/kidding goals. They usually rebound as either anger or depression. That's why Deterrence is the least efficient of the W/L Commands.

W/L Commands in the Deterrence mode are attractive to part-time caretakers and to parents rushed for time because they're the fastest-acting "motors" to stop *mis*/kidding. All W/L Commands in this mode say, "Stop it, (or else!)", where the "or elses" are unpleasant (-) A/L Consequences. The power and effectiveness of these commands in stopping Out/kidding comes from the fact that there are almost no limits to the intensity of (-) A/L Consequences. These commands are also the easiest to "wire." As you'll see in Chapter Five, choosing unpleasant (-) A/L Consequences for kids requires little planning, since most work equally well for all kids at every age.

Remember, A/L Consequences "activate" W/L to make W/L Commands. Don't worry about A/L Consequences now; I'll show you how to choose them and use them in the next chapter. Let's look at some examples of W/L Commands presented to kids to DETER Out/kidding.

Using W/L Commands in the Deterrence Mode: "STOP IT, or ([-] A/L Consequence)

Here's a deterrent W/L Command for a ten month old baby that cries whenever its parents put it down. It's not important that the baby understand the words. A/L Consequences speak for themselves:

"Stop crying, or (we'll leave the room)."

The first time this command is given, most babies will cry longer and louder. The command, including its A/L Consequence, must be repeated and acted out several times before it will be effective; that is, the parents must consistently leave the room when the baby continues to cry. This establishes the "honesty" of the command. After a while, the baby will realize that its misdirected Out/kidding goal of keeping the parents in the room by crying cannot be achieved; rather, it must remain quiet and not cry if the parents are to stay.

Here's another deterrent W/L Command for a three year old hitting its playmates, unprovoked:

"Stop hitting, or (you'll go to the time out room)."

As in the first example, it's likely this kid will test the command and end up screaming in the time out room. The kid's underlying motivation for hitting the playmates hasn't been vented, redirected or even identified. It's been "splattered" against an A/L Consequence, going to the time out room.

A deterrent W/L Command for a ten year old using foul language in school might be phrased:

"If any teachers complain that you curse in school, (you'll be grounded for a week)."

Since the only way you'd know about this Out/kidding would be if someone complained, the command is aimed at stopping the complaints.

Here's a deterrent W/L Command directed at a sixteen year old who takes his parents' belongings without permission:

"If you take things without permission, (you won't be allowed to drive)."

Deterrence, because it "splatters" kids' energies against A/L Consequences, creates anger or depression. These reactions may lead to more *mis*/kidding. Sometimes, if emotions get out of control, *KILLER*/kidding may result. In the examples above, the three year old, in the time out room, may resort to wetting or soiling clothes or even self-mutilation. The grounded ten year old may physically attack younger siblings and the teenager may ignore curfews or even steal a car.

In general, the more effort or energy kids put into Out/kidding, the greater the risk that the "splatter" of Deterrence will work against you in your role as an authority. There are two better W/L Commands for managing Out/kidding that utilize kids' misdirected energies to achieve good/kidding. One of them, Deflection, is diagrammed below:

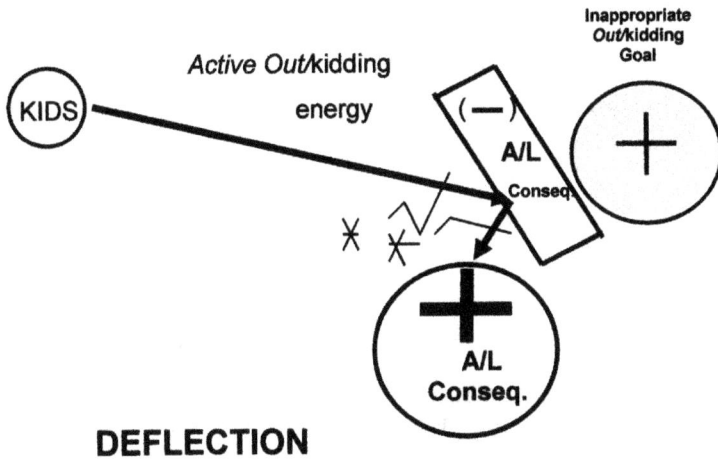

DEFLECTION

W/L Commands that deflect Out/kidding are "wired" to use both an unpleasant (-) A/L Consequence to limit misdirected efforts and one or more compelling (+) A/L Consequences to redirect inappropriate motivation toward good/kidding. Deflection, like Deterrence, works rapidly to stop Out/kidding. Though some "splattering" of energy occurs if kids elect to test the command, deflection preserves most of kids' motivation and energy to pursue more worthwhile goals.

Deflection takes more planning to "wire" because, in contrast to unpleasant (-) A/L Consequences that are similar for most kids, compelling (+) A/L Consequences are different for different kids. Again, our immediate purpose here is to become familiar with the W/L Commands. We'll consider A/L Consequences later.

Here are some W/L Commands that Deflect Out/kidding.

Using W/L Commands In The Deflection Mode: "Stop that or ([-] A/L Consequence); do this instead and ([+] A/L Consequence."

Here's a deflecting W/L Command for a ten month old baby crying whenever its parents put it down. As before, the baby need not understand the words. A/L Consequences speak for themselves:

"When you cry, (we'll put you down); when you're quiet (we'll pick you up)."

In this situation, the baby will cry several times when it's put down, but it will discover that its parents can be lured back with silence. Eventually, much of the energy the baby directed at crying (Out/kidding) will be redirected at quiet play with the parents (Good/kidding).

For the three year old who hits playmates unprovoked, here's a W/L Command to deflect that Out/kidding:

"Stop hitting or (you'll go to the time-out room); if you help Johnny fill his pail with sand (you may have an ice cream)."

For the ten year old using foul language in school:

"If your teachers complain about your language (you'll be grounded); if your teachers tell me you've been courteous this week (we'll go fishing)."

And for the sixteen year old taking parents' things without permission:

"If you take things without asking (you'll be forbidden to drive for a month); if you consistently ask permission when you use our things (your curfew will be extended to midnight)."

W/L Commands "wired" to Deflect active Out/kidding are safer for kids and more energy-conserving for both kids and adults than Deterrence since they cause kids less anger and depression. Unpleasant (-) A/L Consequences can be chosen easily without intimate knowledge of kids' likes and dislikes. The (-) A/L Consequences within these commands Deflect continued Out/kidding even if the (+) A/L components are poorly chosen. When (+) A/L Consequences are well-chosen, they preserve kids' motivation for good/kidding goals. I recommend Deflection as the "motor" of choice for managing active Out/kidding, especially where time is of the essence and your energies are limited.

A third type of W/L Command can be used for controlling active Out/kidding. Diversion, diagrammed below, is best reserved for less intense levels of Out/kidding. When kids are not highly motivated or intent on their *mis*/kidding, Diversion offers a way to move them toward good/kidding without the "splatter" of any unpleasant (-) A/L Consequences.

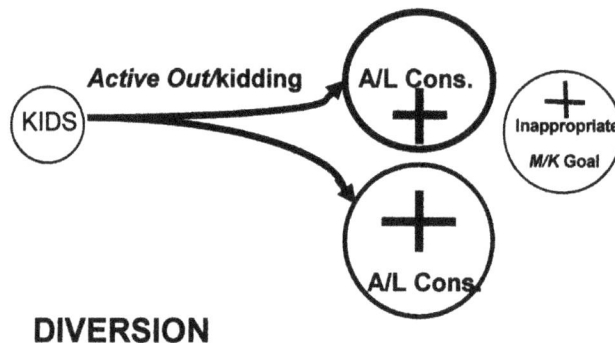

DIVERSION

W/L Commands "wired" to Divert active Out/kidding take longer to work than either Deterrence or Deflection. Since there is no (-) A/L barrier to prevent further Out/kidding, kids will continue their misguided efforts until they discover the (+) A/L Consequences are more desirable than their Out/kidding goals. The weakness of Diversion is that if you fail to select (+) A/L Consequences that are compelling enough, the Out/kidding will continue. Diversion takes patience and intimate knowledge of kids; that's why it works best for parents.

Here are some W/L Commands used to Divert active Out/kidding:

Using W/L Commands In The Diversion Mode: "Do this instead and ([+] A/L Consequence; or do that instead and ([+] A/L Consequence."

Here's the example of the ten month old baby that cries whenever its parents put it down. This time, we use a W/L Command to Divert it:

"Sit quietly on the bed and [we'll give you your bottle] or sit quietly in the bathtub and [you can play with your floating toys]."

This command works only if the parents know the baby wants its bottle or likes a bath. For some babies, one or both A/L Consequences may be only slightly pleasant [+], or even unpleasant [-]. Under the best of circumstances, it will take time for the baby to discover and switch goals.

For the three year old hitting its playmates, a Diverting W/L Command looks like this:

"Help Johnny fill his pail with sand and [you may have ice cream] or tell Johnny you're sorry and [we'll go on the merry-go-round]."

For the ten year old using foul language in school:

"Go to school for two weeks with no complaints about your language and [we'll go fishing]; go for two months without complaints and [we'll go to Disneyworld]."

And for the sixteen year old taking things without permission:

"Ask our permission before using our things for the next month and [your curfew will be extended till midnight]; or, if you prefer, [your allowance will be increased]."

Using W/L Commands to Divert active Out/kidding, though they take more thought to "wire" and longer to work, never create anger or depression. Kids' energies are Diverted to good/kidding goals. The diagram above shows two [+] A/L Consequences, but you can Divert with one or any number of alternative [+] A/L Consequences.

When kids refuse to do things they should be doing at the *Mid*/kidding level, they're already achieving an inappropriate, misdirected goal. From their viewpoint, there's no reason to pursue a good/kidding goal. This is passive Out/kidding. Here, we must create motivation with W/L Commands that Draw kids away from their inappropriate Out/kidding goal and toward a more compelling [+] A/L Consequence. Here's what Drawing

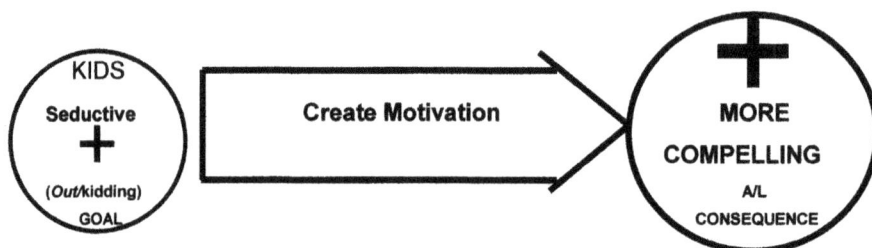

DRAWING

looks like:

As is true for Diverting active Out/kidding, Drawing kids from passive Out/kidding toward good/kidding uses no unpleasant [-] A/L Consequences. In this case, kids aren't doing anything wrong, they're merely choosing not to do something they should be doing. [-] A/L barriers would accomplish nothing and might provoke more *mis*/kidding. If you think you need a [-] A/L Consequence, you're not dealing with passive Out/kidding, but rather with active Out/kidding and any of the other W/L Commands you've learned can be used for control.

Think of Drawing as a form of Diversion where, instead of reaching ahead for inappropriate Out/kidding goals, kids are sitting on those goals. Though only one compelling [+] A/L Consequence is diagrammed, any number may be used.

Here are some W/L Commands designed to Draw kids from passive Out/kidding toward good/kidding:

Using W/L Commands In The Drawing Mode: "Do this and ([+] A/L Consequence)."

For a ten month old refusing to hold her own bottle:

"Hold your bottle and [I'll carry you outside.]"

For a three year old using gesture, only, to communicate to his teacher:

"When you tell me what you want, [you may have it.]"

For a ten year old failing to turn off the TV when finished:

"Turn off the TV when you're finished and [you may watch it tomorrow.]"

For a sixteen year old leaving dirty clothes on the bedroom floor:

"Throw your dirty clothes in the wash and [you can invite your friends to a party here next week."]

Don't worry if you can't always tell passive from active Out/kidding. It's a matter of opinion, and yours is as good as the next person's! Besides, the distinction is made only as a guide to choosing among W/L Commands. If you make a mistake and use a more powerful W/L Command for Out/kidding, it will still work, perhaps even faster.

W/L Commands that Deflect or Divert active Out/kidding and that Draw passive Out/kidding require intimate knowledge of kids' likes and dislikes. This familiarity is needed to choose powerful enough [+] A/L Consequences to run the "motors." Since neither Diversion nor Drawing incorporate [-] A/L Consequences to stop further *mis*/kidding, the effectiveness of these commands depends entirely upon the correct choice of [+] A/L Consequences. Commands "wired" with [+] A/L Consequences take time and patience to use. For these reasons alone, parents (who know their kids best) are more likely to use such commands than babysitters and part-time caretakers.

There are other, more important differences than available time and patience between parents and part-time caretakers. Let's look at some of them. Identifying your goals, if you're a parent, will help you choose the right W/L Commands to promote good/kidding.

Choosing The Right W/L Commands: What Are Parents For?

All kids' caretakers need to control *mis*/kidding. But parents must do more than merely stop *mis*/kidding. They've got to build better kidding; that is, they must promote good/kidding.

You've seen how *mis*/kidding is recognized by its destructive consequences on AGE WORK, OTHERS and AUTHORITY. By contrast, a constructive effect on these Consequence Areas defines good/kidding.

What makes growth in the Consequence Areas so important? It's because kids' success in life depends on achieving self-fulfillment (AGE WORK), getting along with others (OTHERS) and reasonable acceptance of rules (AUTHORITY). But, in my opinion, growth in the Consequence Areas is not itself the ultimate goal of parenting. I believe the ultimate goal for parents is to create responsible adults. Good/kidding permits this process to occur, but it doesn't ensure it. To lead kids to responsible adulthood, parents must furnish three "provisions" for adulthood.

The "Provisions" For Adulthood

Honest W/L Commands

o

Nurturance through love and affection

o

Responsibility for consequences

The HoNoR role of parenthood distinguishes parents from other caretakers. Whenever *mis*/kidding occurs, opportunities present themselves for parents to equip kids with more of these "provisions" for adulthood. Fortunately, the HoNoR role requires less effort than most other approaches to parenthood and it's the most powerful method for kid control.

The Importance of Honesty In Choosing W/L Commands

Cats and dogs are rarely seen ducking their heads in bowls of water or walking on hot stoves. That's because water and hot stoves consistently "speak" in Action Language. Water always says, "If you keep your head in me you'll start to drown." Hot stoves always say, "If you walk on me I'll burn you." After one or two tests of this A/L, it becomes clear to the animals that disregarding it always results in choking or burning. Soon, the animals avoid immersing their heads in any body of water or coming in contact with any hot object. Because this A/L is so consistent, there's never any confusion about its meaning.

The diagram we reviewed of the Out/kidding environment illustrates how parents' lives and those of their kids are more complicated than those of other animals. Besides receiving powerful A/L from YOU, kids are subjected to A/L from OTHER PEOPLE and THINGS. Sometimes, due to guilt, indecision, or lack of awareness, W/L conflicts with A/L. Then, kids must choose between verbal wishes (W/L) and non-verbal reality (A/L). Because A/L consistently portrays the "real" world, it's intrinsically "honest." W/L that conflicts with A/L is interpreted by kids as "dishonest" and is ignored.

As authority persons, but especially as parents, we want kids to learn to trust us. They've got to know they can rely on how we portray their world. They need to figure out which rules they must follow, which they may follow and which they can ignore. Being HONEST with kids is the single most important job parents have - more important even than showing them affection. When parents act "dishonestly" by intentionally hiding difficult or frightening things from them, or by indicating such things don't exist, kids will eventually be hurt or killed. Even when parents unknowingly misinform kids, they run the risk of failing to prepare them to deal effectively and successfully with life. Affection cannot save kids from parental dishonesty.

Most parents would recoil from an accusation of intentional "dishonesty." Indeed, dishonesty with kids is virtually never recognized as such by parents. But the result of discrepant messages from the environment, whether from guilt, indecision or lack of awareness, is the creator of *mis*/kidding.

Some examples of the effects of parental "dishonesty" are worth reviewing.

A Toddler Tests For Honesty: Bobby's In The Kitchen Again!

Bobby, aged two and a half years, watches Mommy frosting a cake. He reaches for the icing and Mommy says, "No! You mustn't!." Bobby pauses. But he's tasted icing before. It's A/L "says", "Eating icing tastes good." When faced with these conflicting messages, one of which is W/L, a verbal "wish" from Mommy, and the other A/L, an experienced reality, Bobby reaches for the cake again. Though Mommy's voice may have been threatening, her words alone do not prevail.

Bobby's Mommy hasn't thought about discrepant messages from the environment, of which she's a part. Her "dishonest" presentation of an empty W/L Command is due to a lack of awareness, but is no less a source of *mis*/kidding, since it is predictably ignored. If she continues to present "dishonest" W/L Commands which are ignored, the likelihood is that more of her wishes will be ignored in the future, some perhaps more critical than preserving the appearance of a cake.

An Elementary Schooler Tests For Honesty: Jefferson Gets A Shot

5 year old Jefferson is brought to the doctor's office for a shot. While he sits on Mommy's lap, she explains that the shot "won't hurt." She tells him to sit still and not to move when the doctor gives the shot (a W/L "wish"). When the doctor arrives with the needle, Mommy clutches Jefferson tightly, breathes deeply and tries to bury his head on her shoulder (A/L messages: "This is terrible! It will hurt. I will try to protect you from the doctor as long as I can. Even I am scared.") Jefferson accepts these A/L messages and screams, writhes and jumps off her lap. He hides under the table. It takes the doctor, two assistants (and Daddy) to hold Jefferson for his shot (Mommy is now in the hall crying).

Besides the dishonest W/L that the shot wouldn't hurt, the whole event has many hidden A/L messages for Jefferson. Some A/L translations are:

- The doctor is a monster who's trying to hurt you (Why else would Mommy run out of the room and cry?).

- Mommy acts like she'll protect you from monsters, but when she sees one, she abandons you.

- Mommy told a lie. It was only by chance that the shot didn't hurt so much. Next time, better to bite the doctor first, before he kills you!

Jefferson's Mommy is acting "dishonestly" through her guilty feelings about having to subject her son to a painful, but necessary experience. The discrepancy between her W/L and the many A/L messages Jefferson receives creates intense *mis*/kidding and virtually guarantees its reappearance at any doctor's office.

An Adolescent Tests for Honesty: Debbie Is Starting To Drink

Debbie, 17 years old, is growing up. She can't wait to be seen doing all the things grown-ups do. Some of her more "grown-up" friends are drinking alcohol. She tries it, too, although she doesn't really like it at first. Mommy finds beer cans in her room. She forbids Debbie to drink (a W/L "wish") and tells her it's not good for her (more W/L).

Debbie knows her parents take a drink or two every day. She's heard alcohol is "supposed" to harm you, but Mom and Dad don't seem worried (A/L message: Drinking may hurt some people, but not us).

Debbie sees a lot of grown-ups drinking. She doesn't personally know anyone dying of cancer or liver disease (another A/L message: If you want to be grown-up, you should drink; no one takes the possibility of disease very seriously). Debbie continues to sneak beer into the house until her consumption of alcohol affects her stamina, her school grades and even her friendships.

Eventually, her parents take her to the Pediatrician who confirms her status as an alcoholic.

Debbie's parents, like those in the other examples, are unaware of the many conflicting A/L messages received by their daughter. In spite of their true concerns for Debbie's health, they act as if they are powerless to intervene as Debbie progresses from *Mid*/kidding to *KILLER*/kidding.

I hope, as you've read these examples, you haven't become discouraged! It's not my intention to suggest that you need to "translate" all the errant A/L from the environment, even your own, in order to control *mis*/kidding. To get kids to do what they're told to do, you need only "wire up" any of the W/L Commands you've learned with an A/L Consequence powerful enough to overcome any environmental influences. W/L, "activated" with potent A/L Consequences and consistently applied become "honest" and powerful W/L Commands.

Ensuring the "Honesty" of your W/L Commands is the first requirement of the HoNoR role you assume as a parent. Tapping into Nurturance to empower A/L Consequences and holding kids Responsible for their acts are the subject of Chapter Five, the last step of the management phase of *MIS*/KIDDING.

In Summary:

Control *active Out/kidding* by choosing one of these *W/L Commands:*

-DETER: "Stop that *or [(-) A/L Consequence]*".

    Advantages-
- Works rapidly.
- Requires little intimate knowledge of kids' likes and dislikes.
- Incorporates only one *(-)* A/L Consequence.

    Disadvantage-
- "Splatters" kids' energies, creating anger and depression.

-DEFLECT: "Stop that *or [(-) A/L Consequence]; do this instead and [(+) A/L Consequence.]*

    Advantages-
- Preserves most of kids' energies for good/kidding.
- Works rapidly.
- (-) A/L Consequence stops the Out/kidding.

    Disadvantages-
- Some "splattering" of kids' energies, creating anger or depression.
- Knowledge of kids' likes and dislikes required to choose the (+) A/L Consequence.

(Continued on the next page)

-DIVERT: "Do this instead **and [(+) *A/L Consequence*]; or do that instead and [(+) *A/L Consequence*]** ."

Advantages-
- No "splattering" of kids' energies, so no anger or depression.
- Preserves kids' energies for *good*/kidding.

Disadvantages-
- Depends <u>entirely</u> on the choice of effective (+) A/L Consequences.
- Requires most intimate knowledge of kids' likes and dislikes.
- Takes more time to work.

Control *passive Out*/kidding with this *W/L Command:*

-DRAW: "Do this **and [(+) A/L Consequence].**"

Advantages-
- No "splatter" of kids' energies, so no anger or depression.
- Creates motivation for kids to pursue *good*/kidding

Disadvantages-
- Depends <u>entirely</u> on the choice of effective (+) A/L Consequences.
- Takes time to work.

To make W/L into a ***Command*** rather than a *wish*, you must:

1. ***Honestly predict*** A/L Consequences (be <u>consistent</u>) and,
2. **"Wire" those A/L Consequences into the W/L to make it a *Command.***

CHAPTER FIVE

Activating W/L Commands: Action Language Consequences

Word Language (W/L) that tells kids what to do is merely an expression of wishes unless it's followed by consequences. In other words, W/L is transformed into W/L Commands by Action Language (A/L) Consequences. When what you tell kids (W/L) consistently predicts the A/L Consequences of their acts, the W/L becomes activated into commands and is accepted as "Honest." W/L that conflicts with A/L Consequences through inconsistency is considered "dishonest" by kids, is meaningless and is ignored. For parents, acting to provide "Honest" W/L Commands is the first requirement of the HoNoR role.

Kids rely on the "Honesty" of W/L Commands to learn about their environment. They know intuitively that this is critical for their survival. Thus kids follow "honest" commands and ignore "dishonest" commands. People often ask, "How can I get my kids to do what I tell them to do?" The answer is: By using "Honest" W/L Commands. In the previous chapter we saw three kids recognize and ignore "dishonest" W/L Commands.

While the first requirement of the HoNoR role is "Honesty", the second requirement is Nurturance. Within its province lie A/L Consequences so powerful that they can overwhelm all competing Out/kidding goals. When Nurturance is employed as A/L Consequences to activate W/L Commands, kids are compelled to do what you tell them to do. Let's look more closely at Nurturance.

Nurturance: Like Honesty, Another Series of Acts

All the things parents do to raise kids are Nurturance. Kids need nurturance to grow. By providing more of it over a longer period of time than anyone else, parents influence kids' growth more powerfully than any other authority persons. One part of nurturance is necessary under all circumstances for kids to survive. Another part of nurturance is not life sustaining, but is simply enjoyable. These "required" and "optional" parts of nurturance are LOVE and AFFECTION. Their relationship is diagrammed below:

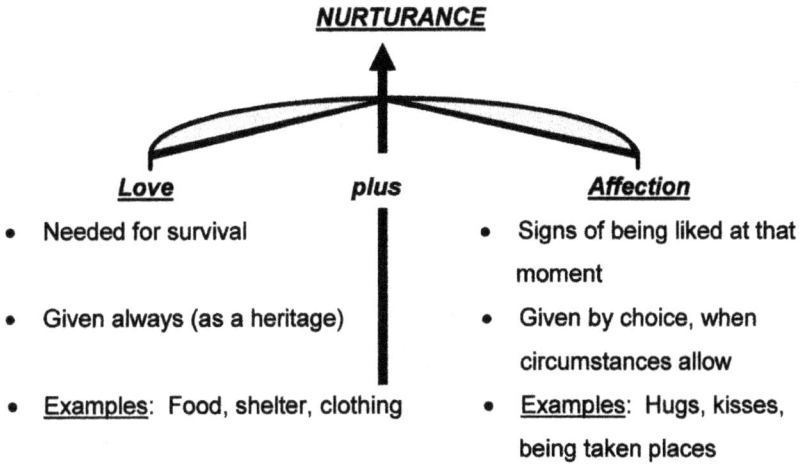

NURTURANCE

Love	_plus_	_Affection_
• Needed for survival		• Signs of being liked at that moment
• Given always (as a heritage)		• Given by choice, when circumstances allow
• <u>Examples</u>: Food, shelter, clothing		• <u>Examples</u>: Hugs, kisses, being taken places

About Love

Love is the life-sustaining part of nurturance. To be an effective part of kids' environment, that is, to have any active influence on kids' growth, love must "speak" in Action Language. This means love can only affect kids through its A/L Consequences. The most rudimentary A/L Consequences of love are the consistent provision of Food, Shelter and Clothing, "no strings attached." Another definition of love is being there when it counts.

Love is a heritage, completely independent of kidding (or _mis_/kidding). No matter how obnoxious _mis_/kidding becomes, parents don't have the right to deny love to their kids. Even when they cannot themselves provide Food, Shelter or Clothing, parents have a duty to provide the A/L Consequences of love through other individuals or agencies. Failure to do so defines parental negligence.

Since love is perceived only through its A/L Consequences, it must be considered a series of acts rather than a "feeling." "Loving" kids is best viewed as hard work rather than a strong emotion. "Telling" kids you "love" them is a non-event. Without A/L Consequences, the words are merely wishes to love. They are meaningless, dishonest and (justifiably) ignored.

Because kids perceive love through its A/L Consequences, denying Food, Shelter or Clothing translates into withdrawal of the survival part of nurturance. This creates immediate panic for kids and leads to major _mis_/kidding. We never deny or threaten to deny love to control _mis_/kidding.

Besides being necessary for kids' survival, love magnifies the workings of affection, the "optional" part of nurturance.

About Affection

Affection is what we give when we hug, kiss, touch, hold, take kids places and buy them things. It's the sauce on the meat of love. Affection alone can't sustain life, but like spice in a nutritious meal, it can create a hearty appetite; the motivation for good/kidding.

Unlike love, affection is not a heritage. It can be offered or denied to kids as a matter of choice. Like any other part of the environment, kids can only perceive affection as a series of acts, not as feelings. "Feelings" of affection are merely wishes to act affectionately. Acts of affection "speak" in Action Language. When caretakers choose to present affection as A/L Consequences, those acts translate into statements of pleasure and enjoyment with the presence and behavior of kids. A message is given that we are pleased by the kids' proximity to us and by their (current) activities.

When we caretakers choose to withhold affection as an A/L Consequence of *mis*/kidding, that "speaks" of our displeasure and alienation with and from the *mis*/kidding.

If kids' caretakers are parents or guardians, affection is transformed into an even more powerful "super" force that can DRAW or DIVERT kids away from Out/kidding and propel them toward good/kidding.

Affection within Love Relationships: "Superaffection"

Parents and other guardians of kids devote much of their lives to the work of love. That's why within such relationships, affection is stronger than it is from any other sources. I call affection "supercharged" with love, Superaffection.

Just like affection, Superaffection can be offered or denied to kids as a matter of choice as an A/L Consequence of kidding.

Superaffection creates incredibly powerful A/L Consequences. For parents and others who care for kids within love relationships, Superaffection has three characteristics that make ideal A/L Consequences for managing Out/kidding.

Superaffection as A/L Consequences:

•Overpowers all other A/L from the environment.

•Can't be "taken" unless parents choose to give it.

•Can be "wired" to W/L to make potent W/L Commands.

If we glance back at our diagrams of W/L Commands that DETER, DEFLECT, DIVERT and DRAW, we'll see that one or another combination

Alan M. Davick

of (+) or (-) A/L Consequences act to attract or repel kids to or from good/kidding or *Mid*/kidding goals. Although, in principle, almost any A/L Consequences could be "wired" in, the most powerful, the most easily controlled and the most effective A/L Consequences for managing *Mid*/kidding are affection and Superaffection. (Super)affection can be offered to induce kids to choose good/kidding goals. Thus, it can be "wired" in to W/L Commands that DEFLECT, DIVERT or DRAW as (+) A/L Consequences. It can also be "wired" into W/L Commands that DETER or DEFLECT as (-) A/L Consequences when its withdrawal is threatened as a consequence of *Mid*/kidding.

The thought of withholding affection from kids creates guilt and impotence in the face of *Mid*/kidding for those parents or caretakers who fail to distinguish between love and affection. The answers to questions directed at the first two requirements of the HoNoR role will lead us away from this trap:

Question #1: How can I get my kids to do what I tell them to do?

Answer: By using "Honest" W/L Commands. By that we mean that W/L must accurately and consistently predict A/L Consequences.

Question #2: (This is asked by those who confuse love and affection.) Will my kids know I love them if I deny them (Super)affection?

Answer: Yes, if they're consistently provided with love, the "survival" part of Nurturance.

Perhaps you begin to see how the HoNoR role provides a framework for parents and guardians to manage *Mid*/kidding.

Nurture Kids With Love; Use (Super)Affection Honestly to Control
Mis/kidding

Within a loving relationship, affection becomes "supercharged." Like affection, Superaffection can be denied by choice without diminishing, or even threatening, love.

Superaffection is Action Language. Whenever it's offered, it "says", "I like you and I like what you're doing." Using the A/L of affection Honestly means offering it consistently to express pleasure with good/kidding and withholding it consistently to indicate displeasure with *mis*/kidding. Consistently withholding affection in the presence of *mis*/kidding meets the test of Honesty. Doing otherwise is a misuse of affection that (dishonestly) expresses pleasure with *mis*/kidding and encourages even more of it.

You don't have to act affectionately to love kids. If you're there when it counts, providing Food, Shelter and Clothing as a heritage, no matter how

103

obnoxious the Out/kidding and how much (Super)affection you must withhold as a consequence, you're acting lovingly. Kids understand this love part of Nurturance through these acts alone. The heritage of love doesn't depend on affection for its existence or perception.

Let's look at some examples of Love, Affection and Superaffection:

Affection vs. Superaffection: Todd Wants To Stay With Grandma

Todd, two and a half years old, lives with Grandma during the week and with his professional, career-oriented parents on weekends. This schedule allows his parents to work long and hard during the week. They anticipate that in a year or two, they'll be able to switch to a home-office arrangement and spend most of their time with Todd. Grandma is a good cook, keeps a spotless home and dotes on Todd in every way. Besides, Grandma has been lonely since Grandpa died. Things go as planned for the first year.

During the Christmas season of the second year, Todd's parents arrange to take off ten days from work together. They plan to take Todd with them on a trip to Florida. In preparation for the trip, they take Todd to the toy store and buy "water wings", a pail and sand shovel and other toys. They're surprised that Todd doesn't show enthusiasm, but as the vacation approaches, they expect he'll be more excited. After all, it's not that often he gets to spend so much time with his parents.

When the day arrives to leave, Todd says he wants to stay with grandma. When his Mommy picks him up, and tells him how much she loves him, he hits her and bites her. Daddy gets angry and spanks Todd. Everyone is upset. On the way to the airport, Todd, who has been completely toilet trained for six months, wets and soils his pants.

Discussion: Grandma has consistently provided Food, Shelter and Clothing for Todd, as long as he can remember. Grandma's been there when it counted, for the falls and scrapes, for the bad dreams, for the coughs and colds. This Action Language is perceived by Todd as love. All the other things Grandma does for Todd, including taking him to the store when she shops, giving him hugs and kisses and reading stories to him at night, are Superaffection. They emanate from her love relationship with Todd. The "love" Todd's parents feel for him are merely wishes to act lovingly, so far as Todd is concerned. He's too young to care about or appreciate the fact that his parents support Grandma with their money.

When Todd's parents offer to take him on vacation with them, they actually threaten Todd with the withdrawal of Grandma's love, the "survival" part of Nurturance. Todd's resulting panic creates Out/kidding. When the parents buy toys for Todd, they act affectionately, but Grandma's affection is "supercharged" with love. Her Superaffection overwhelms the parents' acts of affection and leads Todd to reject them.

Linda's A Pain In The Neck; Mommy DEFLECTS Linda's Mid/kidding With Superaffection

Linda is five years old and her Mommy has to wear a neck brace. Mommy will have to wear the brace for three months. As of late, Linda has begun to cling to Mommy whenever she's told to do something she doesn't want to do. This results in physical pain and mental anguish for Mommy. She gets angry at Linda because she causes her pain in the neck, but she feels guilty pushing Linda away because she fears Linda won't know she's loved.

One day, Mommy and Linda visit a psychologist. He watches Linda's *Mid*/kidding until Mommy breaks into tears. He suggests a simple solution. Mommy will put a "star chart" in Linda's room with a box drawn on it for each day of the week. Linda is given two stars each morning to keep in her pocket. Whenever she hangs on Mommy and whines to be carried, Mommy takes one of her stars away. At bedtime, Linda pastes any remaining stars on the chart in that day's box. If she has a star at bedtime, Linda hears a bedtime story. Otherwise, she goes right to bed. Linda is told that Mommy will be going to the zoo on the weekend, but Linda may go only if she has a star in each box that week. If even one box is empty by the weekend, Linda will stay at home with a baby-sitter, while Mommy will go out alone. Mommy is unsure she'll be able to deny Linda a trip to the zoo if she doesn't stop her *Mid*/kidding, but the pain in her neck and the psychologist's reassurance compels her to try.

Mommy and Linda return to the psychologist three weeks later. Mommy relates that Linda didn't seem to respond to this plan the first week. Linda kept no stars. Following the psychologist's advice, Mommy managed to have Linda stay home with a baby-sitter while she went out herself. The second week, Linda filled all her boxes with stars. That is, she didn't whine and she asked to be carried only once. This week, several times a day, Linda proudly announces to her Mommy that she's "not asking to be carried." She waits until Mommy responds with a hug. Linda is very happy and Mommy no longer has a pain in her neck.

Discussion: Linda's misguided (and painful for Mommy) *Mid*/kidding goal is to be held and carried. At first, Mommy confuses affection and love. She feels guilty about pushing Linda away because she doesn't distinguish between the affectionate act of holding Linda and the loving acts of providing Linda a home and being there when it counts.

The psychologist helps Mommy (who doesn't have a copy of *MIS*/KIDDING yet) "activate" a W/L Command with an A/L Consequence designed to DEFLECT Linda's *Mid*/kidding. Chosen to "deflect" the

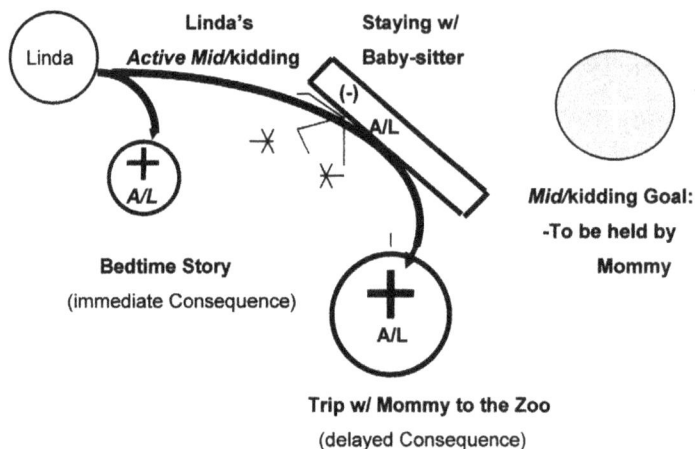

DEFLECTION

Mid/kidding is the (-) A/L Consequence, "staying home with the baby-sitter." Two (+) A/L Consequences are chosen to encourage good/kidding; an immediate consequence, "Mommy will read a bedtime story" and a delayed, but much more powerful consequence, "You can come with me to the zoo." This Command, in the DEFLECTION mode, is diagrammed below:

In the diagram of DEFLECTION you saw in Chapter Four, only one (+) A/L Consequence was shown. Here, because Linda is young, immediate and delayed Consequences are used to insure early success (with immediate relief for Mommy!) and continued good/kidding.

The star chart is a useful "pegboard" on which to "hang" W/L Commands for preschoolers and elementary schoolers. The stars provide incremental reminders to young kids of their progress toward good/kidding goals or their proximity to unpleasant (-) A/L Consequences, if the *Mid*/kidding continues. In the example above, the stars are encouragement for Linda to continue working for a bedtime story. The bedtime story, in turn, becomes an even greater inducement for uninterrupted good/kidding, ultimately leading to a trip to the zoo.

For older, more mature kids who are able to work for long-term goals, written contracts can serve as "pegboards" on which to "hang" W/L Commands. Both star charts and written contracts allow us to arrange (+) A/L Consequences in progressively more powerful sequences to "lure" kids toward distant good/kidding goals. These techniques are discussed in greater detail in Appendix III.

Kids' perceptions of love and Superaffection, the components of parents' Nurturance, are different for fathers and mothers and at different stages of kids' lives. This situation is exaggerated in divorce, where the custodial parent has more powerful A/L Consequences available to "activate" W/L Commands. To successfully control m*is*/kidding, and especially to promote good/kidding, the "endowed" parent must "lend" Superaffection to the other parent or parents.

Here's an example of *Mid*/kidding in a teenager whose parents are divorced:

Mom's Superaffection Helps Dad DRAW Sarah Toward Better Asthma Control

Sarah,14 years old, has asthma and lives with her mother. Her parents are divorced and her father is remarried. Sarah complains that she doesn't like her stepmother (Dad's new wife) because "she has too many rules."

Sarah's asthma requires the regular use of inhalers to avoid wheezing. She's very good about taking her medicines at home and in school. But when Sarah visits her father and his wife, she often "forgets" to take her medication. This results in wheezing severe enough to shorten her visits with Dad. As hard as they've tried, Dad and his wife haven't been able to get Sarah to take her medicines regularly.

Dad, who doesn't have a copy of *MIS*/KIDDING yet, asks his Pediatrician for help on one of Sarah's trips to the doctor's office. Sarah, her stepmother and her Dad meet with the doctor. She determines that Sarah's father and his wife are truly loving parents, but Sarah spends only four weeks each year with them. Although Sarah's Dad is there when it counts and provides for Sarah's needs, for the month she visits, Sarah sees her mother as more "loving" than her father because her mother provides the "survival" part of Nurturance for eleven months of the year. Dad and stepmother's affection is not powerful enough to compete with the Superaffection Sarah anticipates getting from Mom upon returning home.

Sarah's passive *Mid*/kidding is best managed with (+) A/L Consequences ("inducements"). "Splattering" Sarah's misguided motivations against (-) A/L Consequences ("unpleasant" consequences) with DETERRENT or DEFLECTING W/L Commands will likely cause anger or depression. Such feelings on Sarah's part would only worsen her relationship with her stepmother. But where can one find powerful enough (+) A/L Consequences?

After a conference call with Mom and the family, the Pediatrician "wires" a W/L Command to DRAW Sarah toward better control of her

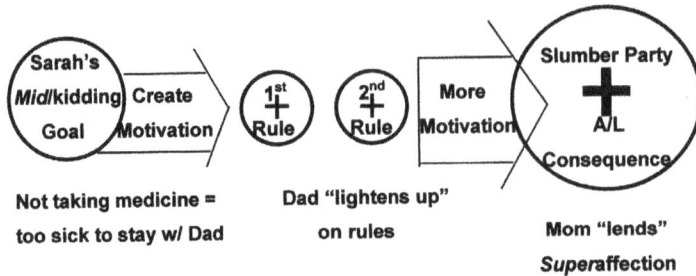

DRAWING

asthma when she's with her Dad. Chosen as immediate (+) A/L Consequences are "lightening up" on two rules by the stepmother that all agree aren't required for "mature" kids of Sarah's age. To make the Command more compelling, Superaffection is chosen as a delayed (+) A/L Consequence; a slumber party arranged by Mom for Sarah when she returns home, if the asthma is controlled with Dad. The details of Sarah's agreement with her family are posted on the refrigerator as a written contract. Here's a diagram of the W/L Command in the DRAWING mode:

Discussion: In this idealized example, divorced but cooperative parents work together to do what's best for Sarah. In less fortunate cases, where kids are caught between warring parents who are uncooperative, only (-) A/L Consequences are available and powerful enough for the non-custodial parent to "wire" into W/L Commands. This leaves DETERRENCE as the sole W/L Command exclusively requiring (-) A/L Consequences. As we've seen, DETERRENCE "splatters" kids' energies against unpleasant (-) A/L Consequences, causing anger or depression.

Parents who cannot or will not "share" the Superaffection of the "empowered" parent, and who rely on DETERRENCE to rear their kids, may unwittingly substitute *KILLER*/kidding for *Mid*/kidding.

Throughout this chapter, the cumbersome phrase, "Action Language Consequences", has been used to emphasize the fact that actions by the authority person, rather than wishes, are required to "energize" W/L Commands.

We've "wired" W/L Commands with either (+) or (-) A/L Consequences, or a combination of both, allowing kids to experience the outcome of their kidding choices. Now it's time to rejoin the rest of the world in its use of more commonly accepted terms for A/L Consequences; rewards and punishments.

(+) And (-) A/L Consequences: Rewards Kids Strive For; Punishments Kids Avoid

I introduced *MIS*/KIDDING by saying there's always a reason for kidding. Sick kids are limited in what they do by their (malfunctioning) bodies; that's In/kidding. Healthy kids choose to act the way they do; that's Out/kidding. The reasons for Out/kidding are always the same. Kids anticipate desirable consequences for some acts and try to avoid undesirable consequences with other acts.

We can call (+) A/L and (-) A/L Consequences rewards and punishments if we remember that "A/L Consequences by any other name are constructed the same." That is to say, rewards and punishments must "speak" as Action Language Consequences. As consequences, they must follow kidding choices. Words alone, uttered as rewards or punishments, are merely verbal wishes and cannot "activate" W/L Commands. "Rewards" given before kids act, in anticipation of good/kidding, are bribes. More about bribes later. "Punishments" given in anticipation of *mis*/kidding (that hasn't yet happened) are abuse.

Rewards are more difficult to plan and take longer to affect *mis*/kidding than punishments. In part, that's because they require some knowledge of kids' personalities and stages of development. Meaningful rewards are different for different kids. Also, kids' attentiveness, organization and intelligence determine the level of success derived from rewards. When conditions like ADHD, Learning Disabilities or Mental Retardation are present, goals may need to be set below age level for age-appropriate rewards. For example, a seventeen year old boy with severe Dyslexia may be rewarded for mastering a fourth grade reader with the keys to the family car.

By contrast, punishments are similar for most kids and are recognized and avoided almost instinctively. Punishments are most attractive outside of love relationships and where time is of the essence.

Some people hesitate to reward their kids for good/kidding. They say they don't want to "bribe" their kids to do what they're supposed to do. Such people confuse rewards with bribes. They forget that all kids who are not sick or insane do what they do *for a reason*. A rewarding outcome is the reason. Here's how rewards differ from bribes:

Rewards Are Different From Bribes: A/L Consequences vs A/L Antecedents

If we remember that "rewards" is our code word for (+) A/L Consequences, then we cannot fall into the trap of offering kids "rewards" to encourage good/kidding *before* their acts have earned them.

(+) A/L offered to kids before they act are Antecedents, not Consequences. Good things that happen to kids before they earn them, or (+) A/L Antecedents, are plentiful in most kids' environments. They include all the loving things parents do for kids with "no strings attached", as well as all the affectionate things parents and others are doing with kids unrelated to their kidding. W/L Commands meant to control mis/kidding must overcome this "background static" to be effective. When (+) A/L Antecedents are mistakenly used to "activate" W/L Commands, they become bribes. They are dishonest, since they neither accurately predict the consequences of mis/kidding nor even provide any consequences. Bribes actually increase "background static" and fail utterly to improve mis/kidding.

(+) A/L Consequences ("rewards") offered to kids after half-hearted or unsuccessful efforts are also bribes, since they don't follow acts that earn them. They share the dishonesty of rewards given in anticipation of good/kidding. Parents often desire to "reward" kids for their efforts rather than for their achievements. This dishonesty can be avoided by breaking distant or complex goals into tiny steps that can be attained and rewarded with less effort.

Here is the Action Language "translation" of a bribe: "It doesn't really matter if you do what I've told you to do. You're being "rewarded" in advance, even if you do nothing or almost nothing, and I'll accept the consequences."

There are two reasons to avoid bribing kids:

- W/L Commands "wired" with (+) A/L Antecedents are dishonest because they don't predict consequences.

- They don't work because kids ignore "dishonest" W/L Commands.

The response to the question, Should I reward my kids for good/kidding and punish them for *mis*/kidding?, defines the final requirement of the HoNoR role. The answer is Yes!, because experiencing consequences for kidding promotes acceptance of Responsibility, which is the path to adulthood.

Responsibility For Consequences: The Last Requirement of the HoNoR Role

Being Responsible means being answerable for one's own actions. Adults are directly answerable for their actions. This is different from kids. Kids depend on adults to take responsibility for their (the kids') *mis*/kidding. For example, when Jimmy swings on the neighbor's gate and breaks it, Mom or Dad, the responsible adults, get the bill.

When kids become answerable for all their actions, they become adults. This is not an automatic process. Many "grown-ups" are still "kids" by this definition. The woman who dissolves into tearful helplessness by the side of the road when her car develops a flat tire is a "grown-up" kid. The forty year old unemployed man who lives with his parents, occasionally mowing the lawn or taking out the garbage, is another "grown-up" kid. These are people who haven't learned to accept responsibility. They depend on others to be responsible for them.

The HoNoR role is a process that "wires" W/L to create adults out of kids. It connects Honest W/L Commands to the power of Nurturance, allowing kids to mature by accepting Responsibility for their acts.

Let's make use of the HoNoR role to apply what you've learned in the management phase of *MIS*/KIDDING.

Bobby's In The Kitchen: Using the HoNoR Role To "Wire" a W/L Command

Remember Bobby, the two and a half year old who's watching Mommy ice a cake? In Chapter Four, before she'd learned the HoNoR role, Mommy screamed, "No! Don't touch it," when Bobby reached for the icing. Mommy's W/L was merely a wish and Bobby ignored it.

This time, Mommy creates a W/L Command to DEFLECT Bobby's *Mid*/kidding. She uses the HoNoR role to "wire" the command:

"Bobby, if you sit on the chair to watch me, [you may have some ice cream]; if you touch the cake, [you'll have to go to your room]."

Here's a diagram of Mommy's W/L Command in the DEFLECTION mode. We can use our code words, reward and punishment, if we remember they're consequences, not antecedents:

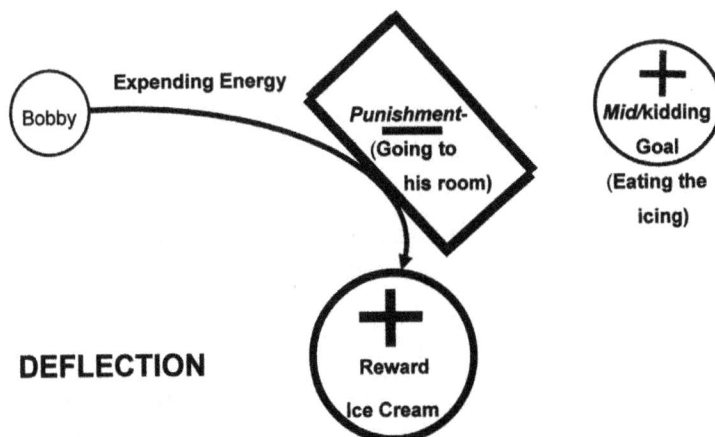

Bobby is presented with an "Honest" W/L Command. It predicts that the punishment for *Mid*/kidding will be going to his room and that Nurturance, by way of Superaffection from Mommy (eating ice cream with her) will be the reward for controlling his impulse to touch or eat the cake. Bobby is allowed to make a choice and accept Responsibility for the consequences.

See now how Jefferson, the five year old getting a shot at the doctor's office, can benefit from his parents' use of the HoNoR role:

Jefferson Gets a Shot: Mom & Dad Use the HoNoR Role to Create an Effective W/L Command

Mommy and Daddy know that five year old Jefferson hates shots. Mommy hates them, too, and becomes upset just watching Jefferson get one. They decide to "wire" a W/L Command using the HoNoR role. Since Jefferson is likely to be angry or depressed after getting his shot, his parents decide to avoid punishment, since it would "splatter" his emotions and intensify anger or depression. They choose to DIVERT Jefferson's anticipated *Mid*/kidding with this Command:

"The shot will hurt like a "pinch" and some boys cry a little. Daddy will hold you on his lap. If you stop crying right after the shot, [you can have some ice cream on the way home]; if you don't cry at all, [we'll take you to the zoo]."

Here's a diagram of this W/L Command in the DIVERSION mode:

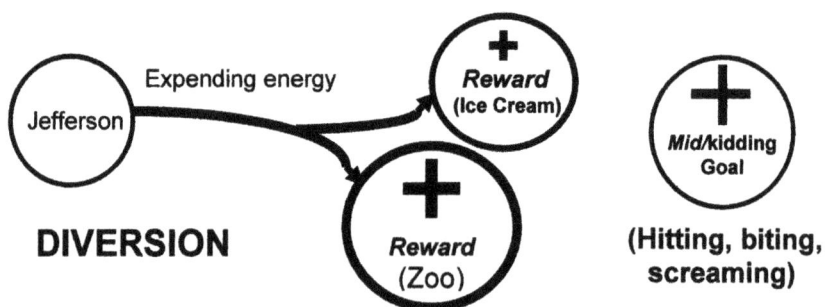

When the doctor arrives, Mommy greets him warmly, repeats the Command and leaves the room. Daddy holds Jefferson on his lap with his son's hands and feet restrained. Jefferson shrieks and struggles as the shot is given, but he's unable to bite, hit or kick either adult.

After the shot is given, Dad hands Jefferson a tissue to dry his tears and reminds him that he can have an ice cream if he can stop crying. Later, on the way to the ice cream store, Jefferson asks if they can go to the zoo.

Mommy tells Jefferson how proud she is that he stopped crying so soon. She indicates that he's such a "big boy" that the next time he gets a shot he probably won't cry at all and he'll be able to go to the zoo.

Discussion: Mommy is totally Honest with Jefferson. She tells him the shot will hurt and predicts the consequences of his kidding choices. She offers Nurturance in the form of Superaffection as rewards (ice cream, going to the zoo). Then she holds Jefferson Responsible for the consequences of his acts. She wisely prevents *KILLER*/kidding by having Daddy restrain Jefferson. She avoids weakening her Command with the conflicting A/L of her own fears by leaving the room.

Jefferson stopped crying after the shot and thus earns his ice cream (the smaller reward); but because he did cry during the shot, he has not Honestly earned the greater reward of going to the zoo. Taking him to the zoo after crying would be dishonest and a bribe.

The HoNoR role works for older kids, too. Here's the case of seventeen year old Debbie. You may remember her from Chapter Four as the girl whose mother had forbidden her to drink alcohol and had told her it wasn't good for her. Conflicting A/L from the parents, including their drinking without any apparent A/L Consequences, had made the parents' W/L a mere wish, which Debbie ignored.

Debbie's parents might have used the HoNoR role to DEFLECT her beer drinking, using the following Command:

"If you continue to act like an alcoholic, with poor grades, diminishing stamina and lost friendships, or if we find more beer cans, we'll have to assume you are an alcoholic, and [we'll have the doctor admit you to the hospital detoxification unit]; if you can get your grades up, stay healthy and resume activities with your friends, and if we find no more evidence of drinking over the next four weeks, [we'll enroll you in Drivers' Education and plan on making a car available to you]."

Here's a diagram of Debbie's parents' Command in the DEFLECTION mode:

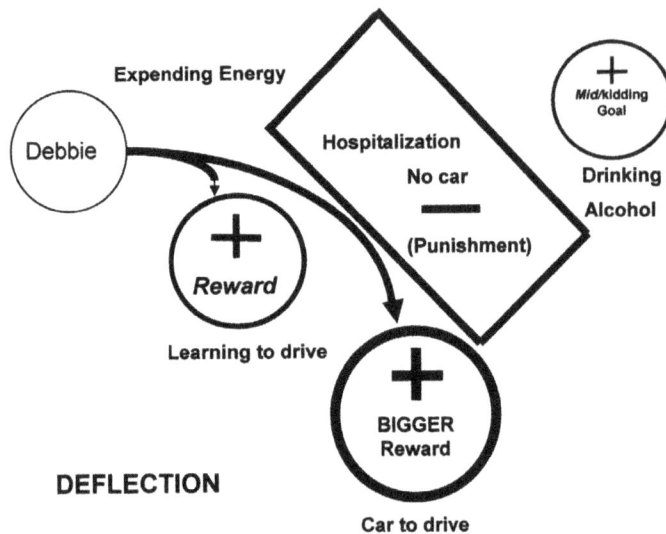

Discussion: Debbie's parents recognize the need to stop what appears to be incipient alcoholism. It's possible Debbie may already be an alcoholic and unable to stop drinking. In that case, she's In/kidding and will need professional help. It's also possible that Debbie is choosing to drink, to look "grown-up" in the eyes of her friends, for example. In that case, she's Out/kidding. One or two "degrees" more on the *Mis*/kidding thermometer will qualify as *KILLER*/kidding and will demand immediate control, with overwhelming force, through hospitalization. For now, there's still time to plan a strategy, but not a very long time.

Anticipating the possibility of In/kidding, the parents choose hospitalization as the (-) A/L Consequence of continued drinking. Debbie will surely see such a consequence as a punishment, but the parents risk the "splatter" of Debbie's misguided energies to shorten the process of managing her dangerous *Mid*/kidding. To induce her to make better choices if she's (willfully) Out/kidding, the parents offer Debbie Superaffection. They divide their Superaffection into two sequential rewards; (1) the possibility of learning to drive, for achieving immediate cessation of drinking and (2) the availability of a car, for continued abstinence. Offering two "stepped" rewards makes Debbie's success more likely since her first successful effort will be recognized and will intensify her desire to achieve the bigger reward. The parents incorporate these Consequences into a W/L Command in the DEFLECTION mode.

By using the HoNoR role to "wire" their W/L Command, Debbie's parents offer her an opportunity to take a giant step toward adulthood.

Whether Debbie is In/kidding (alcohol addiction) or Out/kidding (choosing to emulate her peers by drinking), the consequences of her acts are Honestly predicted by the Command. Her parents Nurture her with love, by being there when it counts, even if Debbie is unable to earn Superaffection. And, of course, Debbie is held Responsible for her acts.

These examples show how the HoNoR role "connects" Word Language (W/L) to the Action Language (A/L) Consequences of rewards and punishments to "activate" W/L Commands in their various modes. In each case, (Super)affection, used as rewards, attracts kids toward good/kidding, while withholding (Super)affection, used as punishment, blocks further movement toward *Mid*/kidding goals. To be effective, rewards must be compelling enough to overcome competing A/L "chatter" from the environment and the lure of the inappropriate motivation for the *Mid*/kidding. Likewise, punishments must be repulsive enough to dissuade kids from engaging in further *Mid*/kidding.

Focus "Wired" Commands On Out/kidding At the Mid/kidding Level

Remember, don't waste "activated" W/L Commands on *mini*/kidding or *KILLER*/kidding. Ignore *mini*/kidding since it's not worthy of your limited energies. Don't attempt to use rewards or punishments to control *KILLER*/kidding. Rather, you must STOP *KILLER*/kidding immediately with overwhelming force, since it leaves no time for reflection and can kill or maim kids or others. Confine your "wired" Commands to Out/kidding at the *Mid*/kidding level. Out/kidding at the *Mid*/kidding level means that kids are making choices that can be influenced by rewards and punishments and that no one is in immediate danger, that your intervention is justified (unlike *mini*/kidding) and that you have time to develop a strategy to control it (unlike *KILLER*/kidding).

Here's a graduated list of rewards and punishments you'll find useful as you "activate" your own W/L Commands to control *Mid*/kidding:

Affection And *Superaffection As Rewards And Punishments*

REWARDS		*PUNISHMENTS*
Allowing an activity to continue	**M**	**Denying or giving some "thing"**
Ex: Watching TV	**O**	Ex: Passing the ice cream stand
Riding a bicycle	**R**	Buying nothing at toy store
Play/visit with friends	**E**	No star for star chart
Driving the family car		Withholding allowance
Buying or giving some "thing"	**P**	**Restricting an activity**
Ex: Earning a selected toy	**O**	Ex: No dessert after supper
Establishing an allowance	**W**	No TV for a defined period
Buy or help to buy a car	**E**	"Grounded" for a set period
(*Super*)affection as an activity	**R**	**Isolation from (*Super*)affection**
Ex: Going to a movie with parent(s)	**F**	Ex: "Go to your room."
Camping trip with parent(s)	**U**	"Eat in your room alone."
More liberal curfew/rules	**L**	"Stay home with sitter while
	L	family goes to the zoo."

Note that on the list above, slapping and spanking are conspicuously absent. One reason they've been omitted is that only *KILLER*/kidding is managed without regard to the anger or depression that typically follow such corporal punishment. Anger and depression provoke either defiance or withdrawal, making the control of *Mid*/kidding more difficult.

Congratulations Are In Order!

Now you're ready to confront the Permissive, the Protective and the Professional Idiocies you met in the Preface. I've paraphrased them below, using the *MIS*/KIDDING vernacular you've acquired. Let's apply the principles you've learned in these chapters to reject those Idiocies:

The Permissive Idiocy

"*Mis*/kidding is too ill-defined to be recognized and too important to kids' emotional growth to be controlled;" therefore "Parents should permit kids to do whatever they please."

BUT you now know that:

> • Chapter One: *Mis*/kidding can be recognized by its effects on the Consequence Areas of Age Work, Others and Authority, and that,

- Chapter Two: *KILLER*/kidding can kill kids and must be stopped with overwhelming force. *Mid*/kidding can harm kids, slowing their progress toward adulthood and must be redirected.. Only *mini*/kidding can be ignored.

The Protective Idiocy

"Kids can't help *mis*/kidding. They're too frail and too dumb to choose among consequences;" therefore,"Parents and other adults should *dishonestly* show their love by protecting kids from the consequences of their acts *with bribes*."

BUT you now know that:

- Chapter Three: In/kidding can be distinguished from Out/kidding. Though In/kidding takes away kids' choice-making, its causes can usually be determined by professionals and kids' limitations can be discerned.

- Chapter Four: Out/kidding can be Deterred, Deflected, Diverted or Drawn to goodkidding with appropriate W/L Commands.

The Professional Idiocy

"Only experts know enough about kidding, and especially about Nurturance, to manage *mis*/kidding without hurting kids or threatening their love;" therefore; "Parents must rely exclusively on professionals to control *mis*kidding."

BUT you now know that:

- Chapter Five: You can use the HoNoR role to "activate" powerful W/L Commands. Affection and Superaffection, offered as rewards or denied as punishments, will redirect Outkidding without threatening love.

- Chapter Six presents a "map" to guide you through the *MIS*/KIDDING process you've just learned as you solve your own *mis*/kidding problems.

IN SUMMARY:

Parents can assume the HoNoR role to create adults out of kids:

- **H** onest W/L Commands are "wired" to <u>predict</u> A/L Consequences.

  O

- **N** urturance is employed to "activate" the commands;
  - *Love,* or "being there when it counts" furnishes essentials and is provided to kids as a heritage.
  - *(Super)Affection,* or the "optional" things done for and with kids, offered or withheld as *rewards* or *punishments,* is made contingent upon *good/*kidding.

  O

- **R** esponsibility for the consequences of their acts transforms kids into adults.

CHAPTER SIX

Drawing It All Together: A Flow Sheet

Now you're ready to recognize and manage *mis*/kidding. All you need to do to solve the most difficult *mis*/kidding problems is to follow the five steps you learned in the preceding chapters.

The first three steps of the *MIS/KIDDING Process* comprise the diagnostic phase. They tell you (1) if you have a kidding problem you need to work on, (2) how much time you have to solve the problem, and (3) if you need professional help. If you follow these steps in sequence, even when *mis*/kidding seems "obvious" enough to skip a step, you'll never overlook In/kidding that kids can't control and that needs professional diagnosis or *KILLER*/kidding that could end your kid's life or someone else's. The process will always lead you to Out/kidding, which kids can choose to control and specifically to *Mid*/kidding, which you can manage with the HoNoR role.

The last two steps of the *Mis/kidding Process* comprise the management phase. They equip you to (4) substitute good/kidding goals for *Mid*/kidding, and (5) motivate kids to achieve them.

At the end of this chapter, you'll find a flow sheet to guide you through the *Mis/kidding Process*. Use it as you would a map in an unfamiliar neighborhood. Though you've just completed a "tour" through *MIS*/KIDDING, working on your own *mis*/kidding problems will better acquaint you with the process. Soon, you'll be skilled at finding your own way through the most complex *mis*/kidding.

Before you attack your own problems, let me draw together the steps you've learned as they're presented in the flow sheet. See how the process is applied to a variety of common *mis*/kidding scenarios.

A Three Week Old Baby Is "Spitting Up" – Is It A Problem; What to Do?

Three week old Timmy has begun to "spit up" whenever he's fed a bottle of formula by his babysitter. He keeps down most of each bottle-feeding. The babysitter is experienced feeding and burping babies. She mentions this to you and says she thinks the baby is "allergic" to the formula.

You observe that Timmy coos and smiles during and after feedings, lifts his head easily when lying on his tummy and is gaining weight and growing normally. Whenever YOU, his mother, breast feed him, no spitting up occurs. Aside from possible annoyance, you're not worried about this situation.

Is this *mis*/kidding? Does Timmy need to see the doctor? What, if anything, should you do?

You might be tempted to jump to the conclusion that Timmy is Out/kidding; that is, discriminating in some way against the babysitter. Or perhaps you agree with the sitter that Timmy is allergic to the formula, an example of In/kidding. Both conclusions lead down twisted paths. Here's what happens when you follow the *Mis/kidding Process*:

First step;

To recognize *mis*/kidding, check the Consequence Areas-

Age Work: Is Timmy failing to achieve normal *physical* development? (You can get a description of "normal" *physical* development in Appendix I). You discover Timmy's *physical* development is normal. Likewise, the *social* and *communication* components of Timmy's Age Work are normal. Timmy's Age Work is NOT affected.

Others: At least one Other (the babysitter) is complaining about Timmy. This Consequence Area IS affected.

Authority: Your Authority is undisturbed. The babysitter thinks Timmy has an allergy. No one's Authority is affected.

Since at least one Consequence Area is affected, you conclude Timmy IS *mis*/kidding.

Second step;

Is the *mis*/kidding *KILLER*/kidding, *Mid*/kidding or *mini*/kidding?

Your emotional reaction: annoyance ("cool") = 1 degree

Consequence Areas affected: Age Work   = 0

   • Others   = 1

   • Authority   = 0

  Total *mis*/kidding degrees   = 2

Recalling that 1-2 degrees on the *Mis*/kidding Scale defines *mini*/kidding, you conclude that Timmy is *mini*/kidding! No need to go further at this time. You can ignore *mini*/kidding.

Suppose Timmy vomited after most of his feedings, whether they were YOUR breast feedings or the babysitter's formula feeds. Suppose, too, that he managed to keep down only a small amount of milk, that he became irritable or that he began to lose weight. These threats to Timmy's physical health might make you Anxious.

The outcome of the *Mis/kidding Process* would be quite different:

First step:

To recognize *mis*/kidding, check the Consequence Areas-

Age Work: Is Timmy failing to achieve normal physical development? Timmy's vomiting and/or weight loss are NOT normal. Age Work IS affected.

Others: Both YOU and the babysitter ARE affected.

Authority: Remains Unaffected.

With Age Work and Others affected, you conclude Timmy IS *mis*/kidding.

Second step:

Is the *mis*/kidding *KILLER*/kidding, *Mid*/kidding or *mini*/kidding?

Your emotional reaction: Anxiety ("Warm")	= 2 degrees
Consequence Areas affected:Age Work (physical)	= 1
• Others (You + Other)	= 2
• Authority	= 0
Total *mis*/kidding degrees	= <u>5</u>

Recalling that 3-6 degrees on the *Mis*/kidding Scale define *Mid*/kidding, you conclude that Timmy is *Mid*/kidding. Although you can't afford to ignore *Mid*/kidding, you know you have time to look for In/kidding (the third step).

Third step:

Isolate In/kidding. It affects Age Work and-

-"looks"	and	"feels"
•Non-selective *		Confusing
•Unpredictable or		
•Of no benefit *		Anxiety-provoking *

Timmy's vomiting, irritability and weight loss are non-selective (that is, they occur everywhere, not just for some observers), they are of no benefit to anyone and they are provoking feelings of Anxiety in you, the observer. You conclude that Timmy IS In/kidding. You must seek professional help before going further. Since the physical component of Age Work is affected, you'll first consult with a Physician, probably your Pediatrician.

When you identify In/kidding, you won't be able to leave the diagnostic phase of the *mis*/kidding process until you've gotten professional help to decide if the In/kidding can be controlled or whether you must accept and live with it.

Let's apply the *Mis*/kidding Process to a seemingly more complicated scenario. See how layers of complexity peel away, eventually leaving *Mid*/kidding that you can easily manage.

An 8 Year Old With Headaches, Stomachaches & Fatigue: Where To Start?

Last month, Ryan, age eight, moved with his parents from their old home in the city to a modern house in the suburbs. For a few weeks he's attended a third grade class at a school in his new neighborhood. Ryan's parents assume that overcrowding at his old school led to his previously poor academic performance. They anticipate that Ryan will respond well to a male teacher in his new class and that there will be fewer complaints from him of headaches, stomachaches and fatigue.

But Ryan's adjustment is rocky. His teacher calls to say that he spends a lot of time "sick" in the nurse's office. Class work is rarely completed and he doesn't seem to have many friends. The parents notice he doesn't bring any homework back from school. Complaints of head and stomach pain are increasing. Ryan is irritable and often "too tired to go to school" at all. Ryan's parents are Anxious and Confused.

Here's a situation that tempts one to think of Ryan as a kid with an isolated "school" problem. If Ryan's parents assumed that, they might proceed with extensive testing by the school psychologist. They might spend time tinkering with Ryan's classroom curriculum. These assumptions might delay the recognition and treatment of a child with ongoing brain damage or worse.

Ryan's parents avoid this trap by following the three diagnostic steps of the *Mis*/kidding Process in sequence. This allows them to 1) focus their energies on *mis*/kidding, 2) STOP *KILLER*/kidding and ignore *mini*/kidding, and 3) recognize and get the right professional help for any In/kidding:

First step;

To recognize *mis*/kidding, check the Consequence Areas-

Age Work: Is Ryan failing to achieve normal physical development? With his constant physical complaints, fatigue and absences from school, the *physical* component of Age Work IS affected. Ryan's failure to make friends DOES affect the *social* component of Age Work. His poor grades DO   affect *communication* skills.

Others: Both YOU (the parents) and Others (teacher) ARE affected.

Authority: No one's Authority is affected.

With two Consequence Areas affected, Ryan IS *mis*/kidding.

Second step;

Is the *mis*/kidding *KILLER*/kidding, *Mid*/kidding or *mini*/kidding?

Your emotional reaction: Confusion ("Warm") = 2 degrees

Consequence Areas affected:

Age Work	
•*physical*	= 1
•*social*	= 1
•*communication*	= 1
Age Work	= 3 degrees
Others	= 2
Authority	= 0 degrees
Total *mis*/kidding degrees	= <u>8 degrees</u>

Ryan's parents recognize *KILLER*/kidding (7 thru 9 "degrees"). The *mis*/kidding "thermometer" has identified it, even though the parents' emotional reaction never quite reached the level of FEAR. Now the parents know the *mis*/kidding must be stopped immediately, but they don't know how to convert it to *Mid*/kidding without expert help. No matter! The third step of the *Mis*/kidding Process applies equally well to any level In/kidding and guides them to a decision:

Third step:

Isolate *In/kidding*. It affects *Age Work* and -

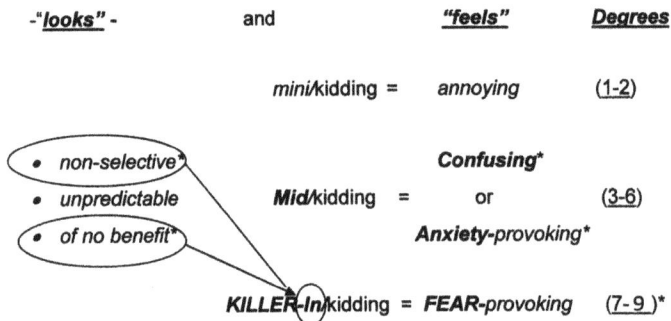

-"*looks*" -	and	"*feels*"	Degrees
	mini/kidding =	annoying	(1-2)
• non-selective*		**Confusing***	
• unpredictable	**Mid/kidding** =	or	(3-6)
• of no benefit*		**Anxiety-**provoking*	
KILLER-In/kidding =		FEAR-provoking	(7-9)*

Ryan's *mis*/kidding is non-selective, occurring both at home and at school, and is of no benefit to him. Though his parents might not recognize this at first as *KILLER*/kidding for lack of FEAR, it generates 7 "degrees" on the *mis*/kidding scale and must be STOPPED immediately. The *KILLER*/kidding has the "look" and "feel" of In/kidding. As with In/kidding at any level, the affected components of Age Work direct the parents to professional helpers.

In Ryan's scenario, all three components of Age Work are involved. All three professional disciplines may eventually be required, but, as you've learned to do, the parents seek professional help in this sequence:

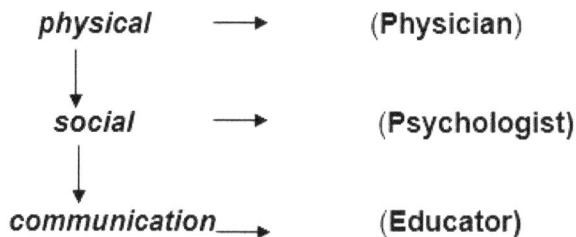

physical ⟶ (**Physician**)
↓
social ⟶ (**Psychologist**)
↓
communication ⟶ (**Educator**)

Ryan is taken to the Pediatrician. After speaking with the family, examining Ryan and performing blood tests, the doctor discovers that Ryan is suffering from severe lead poisoning. He was probably exposed to lead in his "old" home, which is later shown to have flaking lead-based paint. Arrangements are made for immediate hospitalization and medical therapy.

In the preceding example, Ryan's parents discover *KILLER*-In/kidding. Because they need expert help to STOP the *KILLER*/kidding, the parents look to the affected component of Age Work to choose the best professional helper. Since the physical component is affected, a physician's help is sought and Ryan is hospitalized.

In the next example, Ryan engages in *KILLER*-Out/kidding. As with *KILLER*/kidding of any kind, it must be STOPPED immediately. Again, the parents find they need expert help to achieve control:

An Eight Year Old Underachiever Who Sets Fires In School

Ryan is discharged from the hospital with blood lead levels under control. At home, he's active and no longer complains of headaches or stomachaches.

At school, Ryan is disruptive in class. When disciplined, he complains of "feeling sick" and insists on going to the Nurse's office. His grades are dismal. One day, Ryan's parents receive a FEAR-provoking call from the principal. Ryan has been suspended for stealing his teacher's cigarette lighter and setting fire to a trashcan. The principal wants to know what the parents intend to do.

The *Mis*/kidding Process is now all too familiar to these parents!

First step:

To recognize *mis*/kidding, check the Consequence Areas-

Age Work: Ryan is NOT failing to achieve normal *physical* development. Ryan's *social* development IS affected by his disruptive behavior. His poor grades DO affect *communication* skills.

Others: Both YOU (his parents) and Others (classmates and teachers) ARE affected.

Authority: Breaking reasonable rules DOES affect Authority.

With all three Consequence Areas affected, Ryan IS *mis*/kidding.

Second step:

Is the *mis*/kidding *KILLER*/kidding, *Mid*/kidding or *mini*/kidding?

Your emotional reaction: FEAR ("hot")   = 3 degrees

Consequence Areas affected:

Age Work

•*social*   = 1

•*communication*   = 1

Total   = <u>2 degrees</u>

Others   = <u>2 degrees</u>

Authority   = <u>1 degree</u>

Total *mis*/kidding degrees   = <u>8 degrees</u>

Once again, Ryan is engaging in *KILLER*/kidding and it must be STOPPED immediately. As before, the parents aren't sure how to stop it without professional help. They proceed to the third step:

Third step:

Is it *In*/kidding or *Out*/kidding? This *KILLER*/kidding affects *Age Work*

and — <u>*"looks"*</u>   and   *"feels"*   <u>*"Degrees"*</u>

mini/kidding   = annoying   (1-2)

• selective*
• predictable* **Mid**/kidding   = **Anger**-provoking   (3-6)
• manipulative*

KILLER-Out/kidding   = FEAR-provoking   (7-9)*

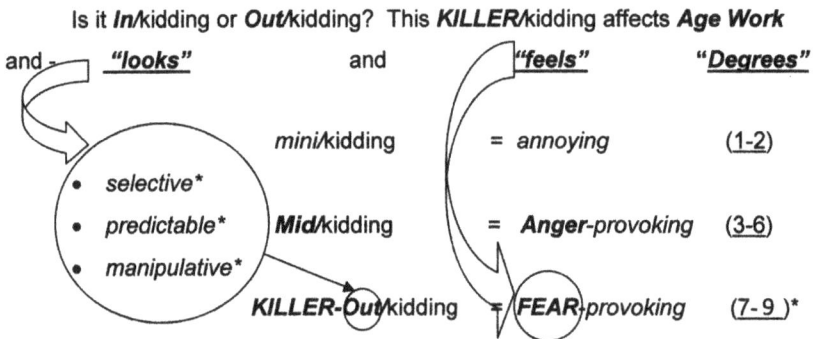

This *mis*/kidding is selective, happening only in school, and predictable, occurring only on school days. That means it's Out/kidding, no matter what emotional reaction it provokes in the parents. In this example, the parents' FEAR generates 8 "degrees" on the *Mis*/kidding scale and thus *KILLER*/kidding is defined. Though Out/kidding is, by nature, willful *mis*behavior, inducing Ryan to STOP this *KILLER*/kidding may require professional help. The parents look to the affected areas of Age Work to find the best professional "fit" for professional assistance:

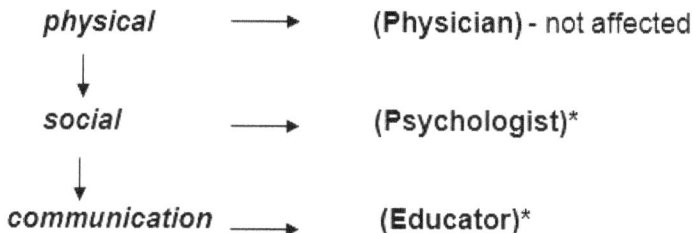

physical ⟶ **(Physician)** - not affected

↓

social ⟶ **(Psychologist)***

↓

communication ⟶ **(Educator)***

126

In this example, the *Mis*/kidding Process bypasses the Physician. Though both the disciplines of Psychology and Educator are affected, the recommended sequence of Psychologist, then Educator is followed and the parents seek help from a Psychologist. They realize that Ryan may need testing and therapy, so they consult a Clinical Child Psychologist. If Ryan's *KILLER*/kidding requires psychiatric hospitalization, the Psychologist will either arrange the hospital admission or later refer the family to a Child Psychiatrist (a Physician).

Ryan begins psychotherapy. The Psychologist determines that Ryan was sexually abused by a male teacher in the first grade at his old school. A long process of discovery and healing occurs for Ryan and his family under the Psychologist's care. Ryan's anger gradually diminishes. He acquires new friends. Though his schoolwork remains below grade level, Ryan begins to attend school regularly.

We'll finish Ryan's story in a few more paragraphs. But first, let's review what we've discovered using the three diagnostic steps of the *Mis*/kidding Process:

First step:

Recognize *mis*/kidding by checking the Consequence Areas -

Age Work: Are *physical, social* or *communication* skills affected? If so, it's *mis*/kidding.

Others: Are You or Others threatened? If so, it's *mis*/kidding.

Authority: Are reasonable rules being broken? If so, it's *mis*/kidding.

<u>Second step:</u>

Define the intensity of the *mis*/kidding, so as to <u>STOP **KILLER**/kidding immediately</u> (if it is present) and not squander your energies on (mere) *mini*/kidding. You can do this by counting the number of "degrees" generated by the <u>sum</u> of the affected *Consequence Areas* and your *emotional reaction*:

Consequence Areas	*Degrees*	✚	*Your Emotional Response*	*Degrees*
Age Work	(up to 3)			
• **physical**	= 1			
• **social**	= 1		Annoyance	= 1
• **communication**	= 1			
			Anger	
			or	
Others	(up to 2)		**Anxiety**	= 2
• You	= 1		or	
• Others	= 1		**Confusion**	
Authority	= 1		**FEAR**	= 3

mini/kidding = 1-2   **Mid**/kidding = 3-6   **KILLER**/kidding = 7-9

If it's **KILLER**/kidding, <u>STOP IT</u> if you can. If you need professional help to stop it, proceed to step 3. <u>Ignore</u> *mini*/kidding.

If it's *KILLER*/kidding, STOP IT if you can. If you need professional help to stop it, proceed to step 3. Ignore *mini*/kidding.

Third step:

Distinguish In/kidding from Out/kidding, to know if you need professional help and which type to seek first. For *KILLER*-In/kidding, you

In/kidding (which <u>usually</u> requires professional help) "<u>looks</u>" -	Out/kidding (which <u>sometimes</u> requires professional help) "<u>looks</u>" -
• *Non-selective* • *Unpredictable* • *Of no benefit*	• *Selective* • *Predictable* • *Manipulative*

will work with the professional to STOP IT immediately. For *Mid*-In/kidding, you have time to work with the professional on developing a strategy to control it.

To find the best professional to start with, check the affected area(s) of Age Work. Use the suggested sequence of experts:

What to Do About An Underachieving Fourth-Grader? - More about Ryan

After a year of intense psychotherapy, Ryan has begun to make new friends at home and at school. He's become a competitive player on a neighborhood soccer team.

One day, Ryan's parents receive a summary of results from a statewide achievement test given to all fourth grade students. The test shows

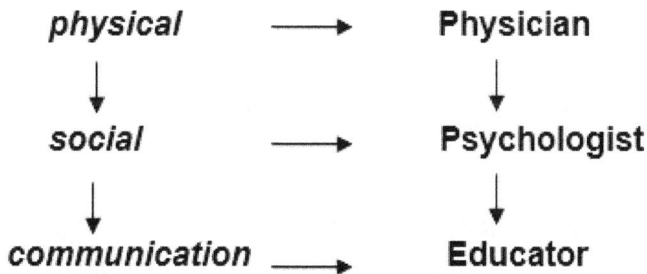

physical $\longrightarrow$ **Physician**

$\downarrow$ $\qquad\qquad\qquad\qquad$ $\downarrow$

social $\longrightarrow$ **Psychologist**

$\downarrow$ $\qquad\qquad\qquad\qquad$ $\downarrow$

communication $\longrightarrow$ **Educator**

that Ryan is performing at an average level in most subjects. In reading, however, he scores just below the third grade level.

The parents check with Ryan's English teacher. She says she knows Ryan is somewhat behind in reading and that she's noticed that he confuses some letters of the alphabet with others. His spelling is terrible. But the teacher indicates Ryan is not far enough behind in reading to qualify for special services. She suggests waiting six months till the end of the school year to reassess his progress.

Ryan's parents are confused. Should they consider Ryan's reading delay a "problem" now and pursue it further, or should they accept the teacher's advice and wait? They decide to apply the *MIS*/kidding Process:

First step:

To recognize *mis*/kidding, check the Consequence Areas-

Age Work: Ryan's *physical* development and *social* skills are NOT affected. *Communication* skills ARE affected by reading delay.

Others: The teacher DOES complain Ryan's reading is delayed.

Authority: No one's Authority is threatened.

With two Consequence Areas affected, Ryan IS *mis*/kidding.

Second step:

Is the *mis*/kidding *KILLER*/kidding, *Mid*/kidding or *mini*/kidding?

Your emotional reaction: Confusion ("Warm")   = 2 degrees

 Consequence Areas affected:

Age Work

•*communication*   = 1 degree

Others   = 1 degree

Authority   = 0 degrees

Total *mis*/kidding degrees   = <u>4 degrees</u>

mini/kidding = 1,2   *Mid*/kidding = 3-6   *KILLER*/kidding = 7-9

Four degrees defines *Mid*/kidding on the *Mis*/kidding Scale. There's time to develop a strategy. But first, it's necessary to distinguish In/kidding from Out/kidding. Remember that In/kidding usually requires professional help for diagnosis and to determine how much of the *Mid*/kidding can be controlled and how much must be accepted, whereas Out/kidding is generally yours to manage:

*Isolate In/*kidding. It affects *Age Work* and –

"looks"	and	**"feels"**
• *Non-selective*		*Confusing*
• *Unpredictable*		or
• *Of no benefit*		*Anxiety*-provoking

Third step;

At this point, Ryan's parents decide to "override" the teacher's advice to wait six months. Having read *MIS*/KIDDING, they recognize that Ryan's reading delay qualifies as In/kidding at the *Mid*/kidding level. That means it IS a problem worthy of attention and though time can be taken to develop a strategy, the In/kidding will require expert help for diagnosis and management.

Ryan's *Mid*/kidding affects only the *communication* component of Age Work. Thus, an EDUCATOR is needed to help diagnose Ryan's problem. Ryan's teacher, in her role as an EDUCATOR, may honestly believe that Ryan's problem is minimal or not yet worthy of further evaluation. Or, she may have budgetary constraints or unavailability of special services in mind. In any case, the parents, avoiding the Professional Idiocy described in the Preface (Professionals know the truth about everything and only they can decide if or when *mis*/kidding should be managed), maintain control of decision-making for Ryan's best interests and elect to attend to his reading delay sooner rather than later.

Ryan's parents meet with the principal of the school and request assessment of Ryan's reading delay. The principal arranges to have the school's Reading Specialist perform an educational battery of tests. These tests show that Ryan has a visual-perceptual learning disability. The Reading Specialist agrees to work with Ryan, using a new computer-assisted program. Periodic retesting is scheduled to monitor Ryan's progress.

Once identified, In/kidding at the *Mid*/kidding level requires diagnosis and treatment. To ignore it, even on the advice of a Professional (Physician, Psychologist or Educator), is to subscribe to the Professional Idiocy. We reject that belief that only professionals can recognize *mis*/kidding and decide if and when to diagnose or treat it.

After successfully passing through the first three steps of the *Mis*/kidding Process (the diagnostic phase), you'll have STOPPED *KILLER*/kidding, identified *Mid*/kidding and ignored *mini*/kidding. You'll have consulted with appropriate Professionals for any In/kidding at the *Mid*/kidding level and discovered if it can be treated or whether you'll have to adjust to it. Only Out/kidding at the *Mid*/kidding level will remain. Some examples follow that show how you can easily manage this Out/kidding using the last two steps of the *Mis*/kidding Process (the management phase).

Sibling Rivalry: Katie and Kristen

Katie, 3 ½ years of age, and Kristen, 5 years of age, are sisters. Lately, the girls have provoked disagreement between their parents and sapped them of energy.

Katie insists on sleeping with her parents in their bed and she shrieks and screams when placed in her own bed. Though she's been toilet trained round the clock for over a year, Katie wets herself when her parents take her to her own room.

Kristen will fall asleep in her own bed, but only if she's rocked to sleep after a story. She awakens within an hour or two and complains of "being scared." Then, she insists on joining her parents and Katie in the master bed where she fights with her sister.

Dad wants his privacy and has tried unsuccessfully to change the routine by punishing the girls. Mom agrees she'd like more privacy as well, but she thinks she and Dad could adjust to the girls' demands. They seem so distraught when they're forced to go to their own rooms! Besides, Mom read somewhere that it's okay for kids to sleep with their parents.

The parents' first impulse is to call their Pediatrician. After all, one girl is wetting herself and the other is having night fears – both "medical" problems. But they decide to apply the *Mis*/kidding Process to see if they need professional help or whether they can manage the problems themselves. Here's how they proceed:

First step:

To recognize *mis*/kidding, they check the Consequence Areas-

Age Work: Is either girl failing to achieve normal *physical* development? Katie IS wetting herself after having been toilet trained. Neither girl's social or communication skills are affected. Katie's Age Work IS affected, but not Kristen's.

Others: Each girl is threatening her sibling and both parents. They and Others ARE affected by both Katie and Kristen.

Authority: Each girl IS affecting her parents Authority

With all three Consequence Areas affected by each girl, the parents conclude both Katie and Kristen ARE *mis*/kidding.

Second step:

Katie-

Parents *emotional reaction:*	**Anger** ("Warm")	= <u>2 degrees</u>
Consequence Areas affected:	**Age Work**	
	• *physical*	= <u>1 degree</u>
	Others	= <u>2 degrees</u>
	Authority	= <u>1 degree</u>
	Total *Mis/*kidding degrees	= <u>6 degrees</u>

mini/kidding = 1,2   **Mid/**kidding = 3-6   **KILLER/**kidding = 7-9

Kristen-

Parents *emotional reaction:*	**Anger** ("Warm")	= <u>2 degrees</u>
Consequence Areas affected:	**Age Work**	= <u>0 degrees</u>
	Others	= <u>2 degrees</u>
	Authority	= <u>1 degree</u>
	Total *Mis/*kidding degrees	= <u>5 degrees</u>

The parents conclude both Katie and Kristen are *Mid*/kidding.

Third step:

*Isolate In/*kidding. It affects **Age Work** and –

<u>"looks"</u>	and	<u>"feels"</u>
• *Non-selective* • *Unpredictable* • *Of no benefit*		**Confusing or Anxiety-** provoking

Mom and Dad can see they're dealing with Out/kidding by both Katie and Kristen. This means they can likely manage the problems without professional help. So, how to go about it? The parents move along to the management phase of the *Mis*/kidding Process.

The girls are doing things they're not supposed to do, the parents recognize *active Mid*/kidding. They understand that Katie and Kristin are expending energy pursuing inappropriate goals. They must choose a Word/Language Command (a "motor" to "wire") to control the active *mis*/kidding. Will they Deter, Deflect, Divert or Draw?

Since Drawing is best used for *passive mis*/kidding, where kids are not doing things they're supposed to do and where little or no energy is being expended, the parents immediately eliminate Drawing. They consider the remaining three commands:

Fourth step; (Next Page.)

Fourth step:

Choose *Word/Language Commands* to control active mid/kidding-

> DETER: "Stop that or [(-) A/L Consequence]".

> > *Advantages-* • Works rapidly. Requires little
> >
> > intimate knowledge of kids' likes and dislikes.
> >
> > • Incorporates only one *(-)* A/L Consequence.
> >
> > *Disadvantage-* • "Splatters" kids' energies, creating anger
> >
> > and depression.

> DEFLECT: "Stop that or [(-) A/L Consequence]; do this instead
> and [(+) A/L Consequence.]

> > *Advantages-* • Preserves most of kids' energies for
> >
> > good/kidding.
> >
> > • Works rapidly.
> >
> > • (-) A/L Consequence stops the
> >
> > Out/kidding.
> >
> > *Disadvantages-* • Some "splattering" of kids' energy,
> >
> > creating anger or depression.
> >
> > • Knowledge of kids' likes and dislikes
> >
> > required to choose the (+) A/L Consequence.

> DIVERT: "Do this instead and [(+) A/L Consequence]; or do
> that instead and [(+) A/L Consequence]."

> > *Advantages-* • No "splattering" of kids' energies, so no
> >
> > anger or depression.
> >
> > • Preserves kids' energies for good/kidding.
> >
> > *Disadvantages-* • Depends entirely on the choice of
> >
> > effective (+) A/L Consequences.
> >
> > • Requires intimate knowledge of kids'
> >
> > likes and dislikes.
> >
> > • Takes more time to work.

Mom and Dad want to stop the *mis*/kidding as soon as possible so they can get some rest. They eliminate Diversion because it takes the longest time to work. But as parents, they want to substitute good/kidding for the *mis*/kidding, rather than merely stopping it and also avoid the "splatter" of anger, if possible. They decide to Deflect the girls' *mis*guided energies. Sibling rivalry provides a powerful source of motivation for this purpose.

For each girl, there are two examples of active *Mid*/kidding:

Katie- 1) Won't stay in her own bed
       2) Wets herself when she returns to her room.

Kristen- 1) Won't stay in her own bed
       2) Complains of "being scared" when in her room.

Each example of *Mid*/kidding requires its own W/L Command. To keep the four examples straight for both parents and kids, a "star chart" format is used. In this way, any number of kids with any number of examples of *mis*/kidding can be managed without confusion. Star charts, like written contracts are simply "pegboards" on which to hang W/L Commands. They have no power of their own.

Here are Katie and Kristen's W/L Commands in the Deflection mode:

Katie- "Stop coming into our room at night, or [we'll put you in your room and hitch the chain lock on your door]; stay in your room at night, and [you'll get two stars.]"

"Stop wetting your pants at bedtime, or [you'll lose a star.]; go pee in the toilet at night, and [you'll get another star.]"

Kristen-"Stop coming into our room at night, or [we'll put you in your room and hitch the chain lock on your door]; stay in your room at night, and [you'll get two stars.]"

"Stop complaining of being scared at night, or [you'll lose a star]; be brave and be quiet, use your 'magic' flashlight and [you'll get another star.]"

These W/L Commands are merely wishes until they're activated by A/L Consequences. The star chart and the stars are not themselves A/L Consequences. They provide a way for kids and caretakers to keep track of progress. By themselves, the chart and stars are empty symbols, having no intrinsic meaning. They are part of the "wiring" of the Deflection "motor" that will become energized only when it is linked to the power of A/L Consequences in the fifth and final step of the *MIS*/KIDDING process.

<u>Fifth step;</u>

Assume the *HoNoR* role to energize W/L Commands:

<u>H</u>**onest** W/L Commands <u>predict</u> A/L Consequences.

O

<u>N</u>**urturance** "activates" the Commands.

O

<u>R</u>**esponsibility** for consequences is left to kids.

Katie and Kristen are told that Mom and Dad are going to the zoo tomorrow. Anyone who has one star can come with Mom and Dad, while anyone with no stars must stay home with the babysitter. Anyone with three stars can buy a toy at the zoo, while anyone with fewer stars can't.

To be sure the girls understand the Commands and Consequences, a star chart is posted on the refrigerator with each girl's picture next to her (two) columns along with line drawings of a girl in bed, a girl sitting on the potty and a girl "being quiet" with a finger across her mouth. Mommy sits the girls down by the phone while she calls a babysitter and makes arrangements "for any girl with no stars who must stay home tomorrow."

Rejecting the Permissive and the Protective Idiocies: The HoNoR Role

The belief that kids have the right to do whatever they please and that the world must adjust to their *mis*/kidding is what I have called the Permissive Idiocy. A frequent corollary to the Permissive Idiocy is that kids are too frail to accept the consequences of their acts and too dumb to learn from them. This I've called the Protective Idiocy.

Fortunately, these parents assume the HoNoR Role and reject the Permissive and the Protective Idiocies. They allow their kids to learn from the consequences of their acts.

It's Bedtime Again for Katie and Kristen

Mom and Dad remind Katie and Kristen of their star chart and what they hope to earn by going to their own beds quietly. They remind the girls that if either of them is unable to stay in bed and needs to have her door locked, she can stay alone with the babysitter tomorrow. The girls go to their rooms quietly.

Things go smoothly for half an hour. Then Katie begins to cry to sleep in Mommy and Daddy's bed. Mommy reminds her that her door may stay open only if she stays in her room and that Kristen is getting a star for staying in her room. Katie begins to shriek and wets her pants. Her parents change her clothes, return her to her room and hitch the chain on her door. Katie continues to shriek and scream for an hour before falling asleep on the floor by her bed.

Kristen, awakened by Katie, begins to complain of "being scared." She, too, is reminded of her goals and consequences. Kristen continues to complain, but falls asleep in her own bed after a time.

In the morning, the family assembles by the star chart. Katie gets no stars and Kristen gets two stars. The babysitter is called. Mommy, Daddy and Kristen go to the zoo, while Katie, shrieking once again, stays home with the babysitter. At the zoo, Kristen gets to hold a toy, but is told she may not buy it until she has three stars.

The next night, the star chart is replaced. The same rules apply, except that instead of going to the zoo the family will go to a swimming pool. This time, both girls stay in their rooms, though both complain till they fall asleep. The family goes to the pool together, but no one gets a toy.

Discussion: Star charts (and written contracts) can be used for successive days and goals and can be applied to lists of *Mid*/kidding problems. They're best directed at one or two problems at a time for the sake of simplicity. Their usefulness and dependability are limited only by parents' creativity.

A Final Word About Out/kidding and the Idiocies

Regarding the above example of Katie and Kristen, parents who adhere to the Permissive Idiocy may ask whether it's all that important that the girls stay in their rooms, stay dry and not complain. But in these examples, the parents have themselves already defined *Mid*/kidding. This means they've determined that continued *mis*/kidding at this level will likely progress over time to a higher level of threat to Age Work, Others and Authority. Providing redirection when required is an integral part of Love (which as you've learned, is usually hard work and sometimes unpleasant), even as Affection is necessarily withheld.

Some parents who adhere to the Protective Idiocy will object to the apparent "brutality" of withholding (Super)affection from kids whose *mis*/kidding disqualifies them as recipients of a reward. They fail to distinguish between Love ("being there when it counts; providing the necessities of life under all circumstances; never contingent upon good/kidding) and (Super)Affection (demonstrations of approval of good/kidding choices; always contingent upon such choices; elevated to the highest and most powerful levels when emanating from a love relationship). Failing to use these powerful "motors" to redirect *Mid*/kidding while continuing to provide affection translates into approval of *mis*/kidding. Such approval may well propel *Mid*/kidding along a path to *KILLER*/kidding and result in more restrictive consequences imposed by others outside the family or even in the death of a kid or Others.

It's difficult for parents to watch kids accept painful or unpleasant consequences, especially if they've been contrived. It's especially hard if parents confuse Love and Affection. But the alternatives of permitting kids to do what they please or protecting them from (safe, though unpleasant) consequences of their acts lead away from adulthood, foster continued dependency and threaten love. Often, to defend against such unpleasantness, parents turn to the Professional Idiocy, a belief that only professionals know the truth and have the power to manage *mis*/kidding. In reality, though professionals can assist with the diagnosis of In/kidding and the management of *KILLER*/kidding, parents, having the power of Superaffection at their disposal in contrast to the professionals, are usually best qualified to energize W/L Commands and control *Mid*/kidding.

The *Mis*/kidding Process presented in the first five chapters of this book, and summarized in this chapter, is a powerful tool you can use for recognizing and managing *mis*/kidding. The Appendices of *MIS*/KIDDING present "Normal" Age Work, More Techniques For Kid Control and How To Hire & When To Fire Professionals. These issues are discussed within the *MIS*/KIDDING framework you've learned and are meant to be reference materials for specific problems you may encounter.

A Flow Sheet For The *MIS*/KIDDING process follows on the next page:

The *MIS/KIDDING* Process   Check any boxes affected:

1

What's worrying you?

Write in the kidding you're concerned about:

Does it threaten any <u>Consequence Area</u>?

Authority……..
Others………….
Age Work
 -Physical
 -Social
 -Communication

(Phy, Soc, Comm)

IGNORE if no boxes √'d.

If *any* √'s, it's *MIS/KIDDING*. Go to *STEP* .

2

Score the "Objective" boxes you checked in Step 1:

AUTHORITY (anyone's) = 1 pt
 You = 1 pt
OTHERS complaining
 Anyone else = 1 pt
AGE WORK: *Phy*=1 /*Soc*=1/*Comm*=1 - Up to 3 pts

+

Now score these "Subjective" criteria – your "emotional" reaction:

Annoyance = 1 pt
Anger, Confusion or Anxiety = 2 pts
FEAR = 3 pts

=

mini/kidding = 1–3 pts → *IGNORE*

Mid/kidding = 4–6 pts → *Go to Step 3*

KILLER/KIDDING = 7-12 pts →*STOP WITH OVERWHELMING FORCE!*

3

Categorize the *Mid/kidding*; it's either:

IN/kidding
- *Non-selective* (Targets anyone, anywhere)
- *No benefit* (Achieves nothing for the kid)
- *Random timing* (Occurs anytime)

or

Out/kidding
- *Selective* (Only some people, some places)
- *Achieves inappropriate goals*
- *Predictable timing*

You will need professional help:
Physician → *Psychologist*→*Educator*
- Be sure to proceed in this order.

→ *Go on to Step 4*

4

"Wire" A *Good/kidding* Command: (remember, until *activated*, W/L Commands are merely *suggestions!*)

• **DETER**: *"Stop or (-) Conseq."* Advantages: Fast; only 1 conseq. Disadv.: Wastes kid's energy, can "splatter" anger!
• **DEFLECT**: *"Stop or (-) Cons.; do this & (+) Cons."* Adv.: Fast, saves kid's energy Disadv.: More work, some anger
• **DIVERT**: *"Do this & (+) Cons.; or do that & (+) Cons."* Adv.: No anger, saves energy Disad.: Takes time, complicated
• **DRAW**: *"Do this & (+) Cons."* Adv.: Creates motivation, no anger Dis.: Takes time, requires POWERFUL (+) conseq.

5

Now, *ACTIVATE* the Word/Language you chose in Step 4. Use A/L Consequences to follow the HoNoR Role:

"H" – Be *"Honest"* by *doing what you say you'll do.*
o
"N" - Use *"Nurturance"* to choose consequences: Either *affection* or *Superaffection* (affection within a *Love* relationship)
o
"R" - Hold your kids *"Responsible"* for the *consequences* of their choices.

Part Three

More about In/kidding Conditions That Obliterate Choice-Making

The conditions in this section are all forms of In/kidding. They obliterate kids' choice-making and must be recognized as causes of *mis*/kidding that kids can't control. This means that the powerful techniques you've learned in earlier chapters using Action Language Consequences (punishments or rewards) to persuade kids to abandon their *mis*/kidding will fail until the limitations imposed by these conditions are understood and accounted for. Trying to force kids to comply with expectations they can't physically achieve will result in frustration, anger or depression and will intensify the *mis*/kidding.

The next chapters present common involuntary conditions that masquerade as willful *mis*/kidding. Though you may not be equipped to diagnose or treat them, this section provides a basis for suspecting their presence and getting professional assistance.

- **•ADHD**
- **•Autism Spectrum Disorders**
- **•Bipolar Disorder**
- **•Cerebral Palsy**
- **•Developmental Delay & Mental Retardation**
- **•Epilepsy & "Behavioral" Seizures**

With each of these forms of In/kidding, you must either change the way the brain works with professional assistance and often medication, or accept and adjust to the limitations the condition imposes to "solve" the resulting *mis*/kidding problem.

CHAPTER SEVEN

A.D.(H.)D.: The Attention Deficit (Hyperactivity) Disorders

What Is AD(H)D?

Did you ever live with an eighteen month old kid? Some days everything breakable broke, every smudgeable smudged, all your tippables tipped. And just when you thought you'd kill the kid, he tried to murder himself! There were times you had to save him from dancing out a window or connecting himself to an electrical outlet. On such days, when he finally fell asleep, you'd collapse amidst what looked more like the birthplace of a tornado than a kid. You'd console yourself with the thought that this is only a phase, that the winds die down as kids grow out of the "terrible two's."

But suppose you had to live with the *mis*/kidding of an eighteen month old kid for eighteen years! The sentence pronounced upon you might be Attention Deficit Disorder with Hyperactivity.

Its Beginnings

AD(H)D is a common problem and affects at least 6% of all kids.

Your baby might begin life with "colic" – rarely sleeping through the night, often irritable, with too much crying. It might stiffen and arch its back when you tried to hold or comfort it. As a toddler, it might not seem to learn from its bumps and bruises, often repeating the same sequences that led to injury in the past. Your kid might be so impulsive or so constantly in motion that you'd be unable to give it much independence for fear something might get hurt or broken. In spite of your kid's sparkling intelligence and promise, you'd start each day with a sigh and a fear of "What will happen next?." You might have trouble keeping babysitters. They'd complain your kid is just too much to handle, though not malicious.

In elementary school, the teachers might say your kid is smart, but "isn't working up to potential." They'd complain of hands that are always in the wrong place; a body that's always falling out of the chair; a kid who never seems to hear directions. When playing with other kids, your kid can't seem to follow the rules. Yours is a kid teachers like, but one who's always getting into trouble.

Can A Kid Have A.D.D. Without Being Too Active?

The hyperkinetic (meaning, literally, "too active") form of ADD is easy to recognize and affects mostly boys. A second type of ADD is characterized by distractibility without overactivity. Distractibility can be considered hyperactivity of thoughts. It causes kids to be very disorganized and impulsive.

Because hyperkinesis affects more boys than girls and is more easily recognized than distractibility, boys with ADHD are usually recognized sooner and more readily than girls, who more often have isolated distractibility.

Kids with ADD with or without hyperactivity can't consistently perform tasks in sequence. They have trouble reaching long-term goals. They only haphazardly anticipate the consequences of their acts. As with all forms of In/kidding, *Mid*/kidding due to AD(H)D cannot be managed solely with punishments or rewards because kids cannot dependably anticipate and learn from the consequences of their acts.

What Are The Consequences Of Untreated AD(H)D?

With either type of AD(H)D, kids will hear, see, feel and smell many stimuli nearby at the same time without being able to focus on any one activity long enough to learn what it's really about. This confuses kids and keeps them from finishing thoughts or tasks. Sometimes, in severe cases, kids will speak parts of two, three or four thoughts at once and be so confusing and bizarre-sounding that some (including an occasional experienced professional) might consider them insane until the problem is accurately diagnosed and treated.

Even when kids with AD(H)D are trying their best to achieve, their efforts often end in frustration and failure. This emotional fall-out can lead to additional *mis*/kidding and, if unrecognized or ineffectively treated, can eventually reach the level of *KILLER*/kidding. In boys, other-directed aggression and violent *mis*/kidding are common spin-offs of long-standing frustration and failure. In girls, self-directed injury, including depression and self-injurious *mis*/kidding like anorexia, cutting and other forms of self-mutilation are often seen with chronic frustration and failure.

Does AD(H)D Aways Cause Mis/kidding?

If kids' levels of activity, distractibility or impulsivity don't intrude significantly (a score higher than 2 on the *Mis*/kidding thermometer) on the

Consequence Areas by interfering with performance in the *physical*, *social* or *communication* components of Age Work, relationships to Others or threats to Authority, this *mini*/kidding may be considered an idiosyncrasy and ignored since it fails to reach a level of *Mid*/kidding or *KILLER*/kidding.

By definition, the last "D" ("Disorder") in AD(H)D confers a diagnosis of *mis*/kidding. In essence, whenever attention deficits or hyperactivity detract from Age Work or relationships to Others or Authority, a "disorder" results. However, you've learned that scores of 1 or 2 on the *mis*/kidding scale (that is, *mini*/kidding) are not worthy of your efforts at intervention. So it is possible to have AD(H)D that never reaches a *Mid*/kidding or higher level. While you'd be aware of a certain level of either distractibility, impulsivity or hyperkinesis, the minimal impact of the AD(H)D on the Consequence Areas of Age Work, Others or Authority, not (yet) reaching the *Mid*/kidding level, would allow you to ignore its unpleasantness until or unless it escalated to a higher level.

In the early years of childhood, it's not uncommon for AD(H)D to be recognized and ignored as *mini*/kidding (e.g.: "He's just being a boy", or "She's always disorganized"). Later in the school years, or even at the workplace in late adolescence or adulthood, as educational or occupational demands increase, AD(H)D previously ignored may blossom into a *Mid*/kidding problem worthy of intervention.

Whenever AD(H)D prevents the performance of Age Work or threatens relationships to Others or Authority persons, it becomes *mis*/kidding. When it reaches the *Mid*/kidding level or higher, it must be treated. It's important to remember that AD(H)D can't be voluntarily controlled by kids without help. While it's true that for brief periods kids can calm themselves by finding quiet cubbyholes or by shutting themselves out of the world in any number of other ways, the energy required for such self-control detracts from achievement and can be overwhelming.

Many kids and adults have tendencies toward impulsivity, hyperactivity and distractibility, yet never reach a level of *mis*/kidding at all. They might be considered to have AD(H) without the last "D."

What Causes AD(H)D?

There are several well-known causes of AD(H)D. Identifying the cause of your kid's AD(H)D is worthwhile because the treatment and outcome is different for different types.

Inheritance: One group of kids clearly "takes after Uncle Joe, Dad, brother or sister" when they were kids. The inherited pattern is often first seen as "colic" in an otherwise well infant. The doctor finds no evidence of abnormal brain function, esophageal reflux (GERD) or other causative conditions in the infant.

It's reassuring to know that in most cases of inherited AD(H)D, things do improve spontaneously by adolescence. If *mis*/kidding can be controlled during the intervening years, the outcome is likely to be a well-adjusted, successful adult.

Injuries to the brain: Another group of kids has a history of damaging events affecting the brain. A very long labor, premature birth, low blood sugar shortly after birth, severe jaundice, low oxygen, meningitis in early life, lead poisoning and many other potentially brain-damaging events are examples. If a previously normal kid develops AD(H)D after such an event, the injury can be suspected of having caused the AD(H)D. Often with this type of AD(H)D, a Developmental Pediatrician or Child Neurologist finds associated signs of damage to the brain. The presence of several nervous system problems together, in addition to AD(H)D, such as seizures, Mental Retardation, Cerebral Palsy or Learning Disabilities, suggests an underlying injury to the brain.

Other medical conditions: There is a long list of medical conditions that can cause AD(H)D-like symptoms, some of which are brain-related and others not. These include metabolic and "gland" disorders, like over-active thyroid, a number of rare genetic conditions (like Phenylketonuria) and certain progressive genetic conditions that cause brain deterioration (like Rett Syndrome or Batten disease).

Most Pediatricians and all Developmental Pediatricians have been trained to look for these problems. When suspected, specialists (Pediatric Endocrinologists, Geneticists, Neurologists) may need to be consulted for a definitive diagnosis and treatment.

Diet: A small group of kids react to components of their diet with typical AD(H)D. The most common additions to kids' diets that cause AD(H)D are medicines prescribed for other reasons. Anticonvulsants (given for seizures), bronchodilators (given for Asthma), sedatives, antidepressants and anti-anxiety medications and in some cases, even medicines for AD(H)D itself can become such trouble makers. Whenever a kid is taking a medicine and having new symptoms of AD(H)D, the prescribing doctor should be asked about this possibility. If AD(H)D is caused by the treatment of another condition, stopping or switching medicines may be the simplest solution. If that's not possible and the AD(H)D has reached the *Mid*/kidding level, treating the AD(H)D as well as the original condition will be necessary.

There is no evidence that sugar causes AD(H)D. Food additives, preservatives, flavorings and colorings have all been shown to cause AD(H)D in a very small numbers of kids. Caffeine, a chemical relative of the stimulant medications, usually improves AD(H)D for brief (minutes to hours) periods, but also results in a "rebound" as it wears off – resulting in an exacerbation of the AD(H)D often worse than no treatment at all.

Except for "eating" medicines, diet is rarely the only cause of

AD(H)D.

Stress: A last group of kids who have no other affected family members (no inheritance pattern), no history of high risk events (no injury pattern) and no association of symptoms with food or medicines (no dietary pattern) will develop AD(H)D because their lives are under stress. Depressed, angry or mentally ill parents or caretakers, drug, alcohol or child abuse by a loved one may be found.

Stress-related AD(H)D is really a kind of childhood depression. It should be suspected and investigated whenever serious family problems exist within the context of AD(H)D. Identifying and treating this group of kids with AD(H)D depends on a careful examination by a Developmental Pediatrician or Child Psychiatrist.

What Do We Know About The Brain Abnormality In AD(H)D?

Scientists think that kids with AD(H)D let too many messages "get through" from outside the body or fail to organize thoughts coming from thinking centers in the brain. Brain cells have been discovered whose job it is to act as a "gate" to control the flow of thoughts into consciousness. These gate cells can develop too slowly (as in inheritance-type AD(H)D), may be damaged (as in injury-type AD(H)D), may be interfered with by chemicals (as in diet-type AD(H)D), or may be overwhelmed with too many thoughts (as in stress-related AD(H)D). An imbalance of chemical transmitters ("neurotransmitters") is one target of medication therapy.

Can AD(H)D Be Treated Without Medicines?

When food additives or medicines given for other conditions cause diet-type AD(H)D, eliminating them or switching to other treatments will "cure" the

AD(H)D.

Stress-type AD(H)D can be "cured" only by removing the stress (e.g.: - a bully in school) or by helping a kid become more resistant to an immutable stress (e.g.:- a divorce). Helping a kid become more resistant to stress takes time and usually requires professional help (Psychologist or Psychiatrist). Until this goal is achieved, a kid may need treatment with medicine to reduce panic, fear or anger and thus enable communication.

When parents and professionals can communicate with a kid, coping mechanisms can be taught to build a kid's inner strength.

Heredity and injury-related types of AD(H)D are resistant to treatments that don't improve the efficiency of the "gate" cells in the brain. Since AD(H)D is In/kidding, it cannot be voluntarily controlled by kids. Word Language Commands, even with powerful Action Language Consequences (rewards, punishments), work poorly and inconsistently. Failure to succeed with these techniques leads to frustration, anger or depression and more stress. These in turn increase AD(H)D symptoms.

AD(H)D improves somewhat if stimulation is removed. Kids with AD(H)D often do better in quiet rooms, away from noise, busy colors and distracting activities. Work spaces with high walls and soundproofing are helpful. Open space classrooms increase difficulty and do not teach kids with AD(H)D to cope with their disability since such In/kidding is not volitional.

What Medicines Are Used To Treat AD(H)D & How Do They Work?

Dextroamphetamine, methylphenidate and many chemical relatives of these medications, both generic and branded, are the current most widely used and demonstrably most effective medications used for treating AD(H)D. They seem to work by mimicking neurotransmitters that stimulate the "gate" cells in the brain, improving the balance of brain neurotransmitters required for successful "gating" and processing of thoughts and actions. Newer medications, like atomoxetine and guanfacine, have also been introduced that enhance focus and diminish hyperactivity. Certain "stimulant" antidepressants are also useful.

These medications work well for immaturity, damage and dietary forms of AD(H)D. Though they may improve performance in many cases of stress-related AD(H)D, stimulant medications often intensify emotion and can escalate levels of "negative" emotion, such as depression, anger and anxiety. Anti-anxiety medications are often a better first step in treating stress-related AD(H)D where the stress is immutable, later followed by concomitant stimulant therapy.

Many other agents are available to treat AD(H)D as either an isolated condition or as part of a group of In/kidding disorders. Some of these medications have more than one effect and can treat two or more disorders simultaneously. One example is an older drug, imipramine, which is sometimes used to control bedwetting, anxiety, depression and ADD, all together. Others are lithium and guanfacine, used for certain forms of Bipolar Disorder, ADHD and Depression.

Occasionally, side effects encountered using a drug for one condition can be useful in treating a coexistent condition. For example, dextroamphetamine, while improving AD(H)D, may decrease appetite and result in weight loss in a child also suffering from obesity.

The scientific use of powerful medications to treat AD(H)D and coexistent disorders in kids requires a physician with Pediatric training and additional training in Developmental or Child Psychiatric medicine. Skillful and effective management of AD(H)D employing these medications, especially in combination, is best achieved under the care of a professional with appropriate training and years of experience. As a parent, one must always assess both the training and experience of a potential "professional manager" of AD(H)D before committing a kid's AD(H)D treatment to that professional.

Here follow some issues to consider before making such a commitment:

Who's Responsible For Recognizing AD(H)D?

AD(H)D can first be recognized as a problem worth doing something about when it results in *Mid*/kidding (or worse). Though the *mis*/kidding may not be recognized as AD(H)D at this stage, or conversely, may be suspected of being AD(H)D while actually being another "masquerading" condition (such as hyperthyroidism, lead poisoning, Bipolar Disorder, etc), its identification as *mis*/kidding, its classification as *Mid*/kidding (or even *KILLER*/kidding) and its characterization as In/kidding can be achieved by anyone familiar with the *Mis*/kidding Process as outlined in the previous chapters of this book. This includes professionals, parents or even kids themselves.

Once In/kidding at the *Mid*/kidding level has been identified, professional assistance is sought for definitive diagnosis and treatment, in the following order:

Physician ⟶ Psychologist ⟶ Educator

What Physicians Do For AD(H)D

Physicians begin by reviewing the family's history of medical conditions to identify risks. They must rule out any process that might cause ongoing damage, such as brain degeneration, lead poisoning or an overactive thyroid gland. Medicines taken for other reasons may contribute to or even cause AD(H)D. Associated neurological conditions, like Tourette Disorder, Cerebral Palsy or Epilepsy and associated psychiatric disorders, like Bipolar Disorder, need to be identified and treated.

The doctor may next gather observations from teachers and family members to compare kids' behaviors in different settings. This should confirm the "non-selective" nature of the In/kidding and may help categorize the type of AD(H)D present.

Physical and neurological examinations usually follow. Laboratory tests may be performed. It is at this point that conditions masquerading as AD(H)D will be recognized.

After the *physical* component of Age Work has been assessed by the Physician, any threats to the *social* component of Age Work need to be evaluated by a Psychologist.

What Psychologists Do For AD(H)D

Psychologists measure levels of ability in the many areas of "intelligence", the degree to which achievement of age-appropriate skills has occurred, the intensity and healthfulness of emotionality, and the extent to which kids can understand and accept limits.

After ability, achievement levels, emotionality and comprehension and acceptance of limits have been measured and compared to norms, experienced Child Psychologists help parents, teachers and physicians understand a kid's intellectual strengths, learning styles, perceptions and self-esteem and interpersonal skills. These measures form the basis for reasonable parental expectations and educational goals; that is, that kid's good/kidding goals. These measures provide us with the proper "words" to insert into our Word Language Commands.

In order to create or increase kids' susceptibility to effective Action Language Consequences that will "activate" Word Language Commands for good/kidding, some kids may require psychotherapy. Others may need treatment for previously unrecognized Depression. Still others will benefit from family therapy. As distinct from Child Psychologists (no M.D. degree), Child Psychiatrists (with M.D. degree) are best consulted when medication and/or psychiatric hospitalization is part of the therapy.

Most kids with AD(H)D find it difficult or impossible to achieve consistently at the true level of their ability as determined by psychological testing. This discrepancy in the *communication* area of Age Work next requires the intervention of Educators.

What Educators Do For AD(H)D

Classroom teachers spend more time with kids than any other professionals, and occasionally more time with them than their parents!

Teachers' observations are extremely valuable, both in judging the severity of AD(H)D and in weighing the effects of treatment on an ongoing basis.

AD(H)D may affect only one area of learning, such as math, or may affect many areas of learning. Additionally, AD(H)D is often associated with other disabilities, such as speech and language disorders, emotional disorders and intellectual limitation. The entire spectrum of learning problems associated with AD(H)D can be measured, at no expense to parents, by Educators. Here's a list of Educators who assess and plan curricula for kids with AD(H)D and associated disabilities:

•Speech and Language Clinicians and Speech Pathologists help kids overcome unintelligible speech and problems understanding and communicating verbal concepts.

•Special Education Teachers help kids acquire and utilize information with techniques that compensate for their disabilities.

•Perceptual Motor Specialists help kids use their bodies to develop self-help skills, communicate their desires and demonstrate their abilities.

•School Psychologists track kids' academic and emotional progress, perform tests for comparison to norms and previous levels of achievement and help design Individualized Educational Programs (I.E.P.'s)

•Pupil Personnel Workers assess the strengths and vulnerabilities of kids and their families, helping them to adjust to disabilities and achieve good/kidding goals.

Test-Taking And AD(H)D

Psychologists and Educators often first suspect AD(H)D in kids when they observe discrepancies between levels of performance in "real life" and on timed tests. Kids who communicate well with professionals in non-test situations, where the rate of performance is under kids' control, and perform poorly when forced to organize their thinking and perform quickly within defined frames of time, are merely exhibiting the very involuntary diagnostic components of AD(H)D.

Inefficient test-taking and disorganization of thoughts cannot be volitionally controlled by kids with AD(H)D, even though they may possess the required knowledge and skills demanded by the tests. For kids with AD(H)D, separating the test-taking process from the content of the tests is critical to measuring true mastery of the knowledge and skills in question. For this reason, an important service professionals can provide for kids with AD(H)D is to document the condition and allow for the taking of untimed tests.

Remember The Difference Between "Disorder" and "Disability!

"Disorders", like AD(H)D do not inevitably lead to "disability." A disorder, though ultimately defined by professionals in mathematical terms, can best be viewed as a significant "difference" an individual displays in measured ability from the "norm." Depending on the environment and its demands, the disorder will reach the level of a "disability" only if required tasks cannot be performed. In some environments, a disorder leads to major disability while in others, the disorder is not even suspected. Viewed through the *Mis*/kidding Process, a disorder reaches the level of a disability only when poor performance reaches a level of *Mid*/kidding or *KILLER*/kidding.

An example may be helpful. If you were an Australian aborigine and had the misfortune to be unable to detect the presence of water in the wind, as the "normal" aborigine is able to do, you might be diagnosed in Australia as having a "WDD" (Water Detection Disability"). On the Australian plains, this would soon be recognized by readers of *MIS*/KIDDING as *mis*/kidding at the *KILLER*/kidding level, since it might lead to death! The "disorder" would clearly reach the level of a "disability." In another environment, such as New York City where water fountains abound, both the disorder and the disability would be unsuspected, there being no observed "*mis*/kidding." Yet even on the Australian plain, the disability could be eliminated, though not the disorder, by providing the individual with a humidity-detecting instrument.

Just as the person with a "WDD" on the Australian plain might compensate for the disorder with a water detector and avoid "disability", individuals with AD(H)D can compensate for their disorder using organizational aids, quiet cubby-holes to work in or medications to avoid "disability."

When Can We Stop Treating AD(H)D?

Though only Physicians prescribe medicines for AD(H)D, Psychologists determine intellectual ability and Educators develop curricula, the responsibility for managing and deciding when to stop managing AD(H)D is shared by each person affected by the consequences of the *mis*/kidding, including the kid. The ultimate decision to treat or not treat AD(H)D falls not with professionals (see the Professional Idiocy in the Preface), but with families familiar with the *Mis*/kidding Process and the concept of *mini*/kidding.

CHAPTER EIGHT

AUTISTIC SPECTRUM DISORDERS

What Are Autistic Spectrum Disorders (ASD)?

Autistic Spectrum Disorders are a group of In/kidding conditions beginning in early childhood and characterized by one or more of the following impairments:

- Trouble relating to Others, as for example –

    o Inability to "read" people's body language

    o Inability to make friends

    o Inability to share or express feelings

- Trouble communicating to Others, as for example –

    o Speech delays or even the failure to develop speech

    o Inability to "make believe" or play at age appropriate levels

    o Strange or limited choices of speech

- Preoccupation with limited areas of interest, as for example –

    o Relating to one or more parts of an object or person, rather than the "whole"

    o Engaging in repetitive routines seemingly unrelated to the circumstances

When all three areas of impairment listed above begin to appear before the age of three years, the most likely diagnosis will be one or another form of "Autism" [1]. Autism may exist along with other forms of In/kidding, such as ADHD, Bipolar Disorder, Cerebral Palsy, Developmental Delay, Mental Retardation or Epilepsy.

Less severe forms of Autism, in which speech is normal, language skills less or unimpaired and intelligence normal or even above average, are often called "Asperger Disorder."

Finally, "autistic-like" conditions, in which strict criteria for one or another of the above-mentioned disorders are missing, may be termed "Pervasive Developmental Disorders."

In all forms of ASD, disturbances in the *communication* and *social* skill areas of Age Work result in a kid's inability to relate to Others and often threaten Authority relationships as well.

How Common Are ASD's?

Over the past several decades, the recognition of kids with ASD's has occurred earlier and more frequently. The estimated incidence of ASD's has risen from about 1 in 2500 kids when Autism was first described to current "guesstimates" of as many as 1 in 100 affected [2, 3].

What Causes ASD's?

There are many theories as to why the apparent incidence of ASD's has been rising since the first descriptions Autism were published. Recently, attention has been focused on vaccines and the mercury-containing preservatives used in many vaccines to stabilize them. The measles and chickenpox viruses, both the wild forms and the weakened vaccine forms, have been suspected of causing Autism.

Heavy metals such as mercury can cause Autistic-like symptoms by injuring brain cells. Early in the course of such poisoning, symptoms may be improved by treatments that reduce concentrations of the toxic substance. Later, permanent damage remains. As to whether the concentrations of mercury found in vaccine preservatives can reach poisonous levels, controversy still exists. In spite of physicians' repeated reassurances that these vaccines are safe, some parents continue to fear a possible causal relationship to Autism. In response to these concerns, Pediatricians now offer mercury-free vaccines as an alternative to the standard vaccines.

Some components of the spectrum of Autistic Disorders are clearly caused by genetic conditions, such as Fragile X Syndrome and Rett Syndrome. These X chromosome disorders can present symptoms suggestive of classic Autism. As time passes, characteristic features of Rett syndrome, such as the loss of previously acquired skills and odd movements of the hands, arouse suspicion of its presence. Genetic testing confirms the diagnosis of either syndrome. Many other genetic conditions have been discovered to include autistic features.

Another condition that presents many features suggestive of Autism, but also progresses with the loss of previously acquired skills by 2 years of age is Childhood Disintegrative Disorder ("Hellers Syndrome"). Unlike Fragile X and Rett Syndromes, the cause of this disorder remains unknown.

No convincing cause for most ASD's has yet been discovered. One can safely conclude that there are many causes for ASD's, some of which may be reversible, others not. Because some forms of ASD's are caused by processes that are reversible and also because effective intervention within the medical, psychological and educational areas can improve the chances for such kids to lead independent and joyful lives, early recognition of these conditions is critical.

Do ASD's Always Cause Mis/kidding?

If kids' can 1) get things done at a level commensurate with their abilities; that is, perform the *physical, social* and *communication* components of Age Work, 2) get along with Others; that is, derive benefit from relationships while avoiding complaints from Others and 3) relate reasonably to persons in Authority; that is, follow rules, they will avoid a score higher than 2 on the *mis*/kidding thermometer. To you, adept as you are with the *Mis*/kidding Process, this low score will merely qualify as *mini*/kidding, an idiosyncrasy unworthy of your intervention.

To qualify as a Disorder through the *MIS*/KIDDING lens, any form of Autism must generate at least a score of 2. Though kids with scores less than 2 on the scale may appear "odd" at times, they will function satisfactorily in all areas of life and require no special assistance.

Who's Responsible For Recognizing ASD's ?

An ASD can first be recognized as a problem worth doing something about when it results in *Mid*/kidding (or worse). Though the *mis*/kidding may not be defined as an ASD at this stage, or conversely, may be suspected of being an ASD while actually being another "masquerading" condition (such as hypothyroidism, lead poisoning, Tuberous Sclerosis, etc), its identification as *mis*/kidding, its classification as *Mid*/kidding (or even *KILLER*/kidding) and its characterization as In/kidding can be achieved by anyone familiar with the *Mis*/kidding Process as outlined in the previous chapters of this book. This includes professionals, parents or even kids themselves.

How Early Can ASD's Be Recognized?

By eighteen months of age, normal kids can demonstrate involvement in and enjoyment of the social skill area of Age Work. When this skill area is deficient, most observers will recognize a form of *mis*/kidding. The unusual pattern of *mis*/kidding suggestive of ASD's are well summarized in the following table, adapted from info@firstsigns.org, (based on the work of Wetherby A. Woods, J. Allen, L. Cleary, J. Dickinson, H. Lord, C.)[4]:

Red Flags of Autism Spectrum Disorders:[5]

Impairment in *Social* Interaction:

- Lack of appropriate eye gaze
- Lack of warm, joyful expressions
- Lack of sharing interest or enjoyment
- Lack of response to name

Impairment in *Communication*:

- Lack of showing gestures
- Lack of coordination of nonverbal communication
- Unusual prosody (little variation in pitch, odd intonation, irregular rhythm, unusual voice quality)

Repetitive Behaviors & Restricted Interests:

- Repetitive movements with objects
- Repetitive movements or posturing of body, arms, hands, or fingers

Once In/kidding at the *Mid*/kidding level has been identified, professional assistance is sought for definitive diagnosis and treatment, in the following order:

Physician ⟶ Psychologist ⟶ Educator

What Physicians, Including Child Neurologists & Psychiatrists Do for ASD's

Physicians begin by reviewing the family's history of medical conditions to identify risks. They must rule out any process that might cause ongoing damage, such as brain degeneration, lead poisoning or an underactive thyroid gland. Neurological conditions, like Epilepsy and Tuberous Sclerosis as well as psychiatric disorders, like Bipolar Disorder and Schizophrenia, need to be identified and treated.

The doctor may next gather observations from teachers and family members to compare kids' behaviors in different settings. This should confirm the "non-selective" nature of In/kidding and may help categorize the type of ASD present.

Physical and neurological examinations usually follow. Laboratory tests may be required to identify specific conditions, like Fragile X or Rett Syndromes. It is at this point that conditions associated with ASD's will be recognized.

After the physical component of Age Work has been assessed by a Physician, a kid's degree of competence within the *social* skill area of Age Work needs to be evaluated by a Psychologist.

What Do Psychologists Do For ASD's ?

Psychologists determine the capabilities of kids with ASD's. Critical testing by the Psychologist includes IQ, Achievement and Social Maturity assessments which build the foundation for parents' and Educators' expectations for the kid at home, in school and in life situations in general. A school's Individualized Education Program (IEP) must be based on specific needs, strengths and weaknesses. Without this testing, there is no way to know if satisfactory progress is being made with whatever strategies are devised for treatment. Ultimately, a kid's ability to live independently as an adult will be determined by such measures.

Psychologists also provide counseling for kids to acquire critical social skills for independent life. Such counseling may be ongoing for many years and often includes group sessions in and out of school for older kids.

What Do Educators Do For ASD's?

Because classroom teachers spend more time with kids than any other professionals, teachers' observations are extremely valuable in judging the severity of the social and communication deficits of ASD's. As the various strategies and interventions of physicians and psychologists are applied to ASD's, educators are perfectly positioned, along with parents, to weigh the effects of treatment on an ongoing basis.

An ASD may have only a mild impact on a kid's performance, as with high functioning Asperger Disorder, or may be severe enough to preclude independent living, as in more disabling forms of ASD's like Rett Syndrome or Autism in combination with other disorders like Mental Retardation, Bipolar Disorder, Cerebral Palsy or Epilepsy.

ASD's often co-exist with other conditions, such as speech and language disorders, emotional disorders and intellectual limitation. The entire spectrum of learning problems associated with ASD's can be measured, at no expense to parents, by Educators. Here's a list of Educators who assess and plan curricula for kids with ASD's and associated disorders:

• Speech and Language Clinicians and Speech Pathologists help kids overcome unintelligible speech and problems understanding and communicating verbal concepts.

• Special Education Teachers help kids acquire and utilize information with techniques that compensate for their disorders.

• Perceptual Motor Specialists help kids use their bodies to develop self-help skills, communicate their desires and demonstrate their abilities.

• School Psychologists track kids' academic and emotional progress, perform tests for comparison to norms and previous levels of achievement and help design Individualized Educational Programs (I.E.P.'s)

• Pupil Personnel Workers assess the strengths and vulnerabilities of kids and their families, helping them to adjust to their disorders and achieve good/kidding goals.

Remember The Difference Between "Disorder" and "Disability!

"Disorders", like ASD's do not inevitably lead to "disability." A disorder, though ultimately defined by professionals, can best be viewed as a significant "difference" an individual displays in measured ability from the "norm." Depending on the environment and its demands, the disorder will reach the level of a "disability" only if required tasks cannot be performed. In some environments, a disorder leads to major disability while in others, the disorder is not even suspected. Viewed through the *Mis*/kidding Process, a disorder reaches the level of a disability only when poor performance reaches a level of *Mid*/kidding or *KILLER*/kidding.

Here's an example of a typical ASD causing disability.

Johnny, 5 years of age, is enrolled in Kindergarten at a local public school. On the first day of school, he comes to class wearing his overcoat and is noticed to stand in a corner of the room and twirl while making odd noises. The teacher, trying to make him comfortable, attempts to remove his coat and hang it up. As she approaches, Johnny begins to screech, curls up under a chair and bites at anyone approaching him. Johnny's parent is called to the school to take him home.

Johnny's parents have had to move several times in the past two years and, although they have been aware of Johnny's strange behaviors, they have not seen a Pediatrician since Johnny received his eighteen month shots. Now, with the school's prompting, they take Johnny to a Pediatrician.

The Pediatrician determines that Johnny is physically healthy. Allowed to play in his mother's presence, Johnny exhibits no eye-to-eye contact with either the doctor or his mother, though if she leaves the room,

Johnny immediately begins a high-pitched screeching. When Mom returns, Johnny grabs her hand and rubs each of her fingers in sequence, repeating this routine over and over as he calms down. Johnny is able to take off his clothes, copy a circle and wash his hands. He is often heard to say, "You go there", though he does not point while saying this and does not direct his gaze at anyone while speaking. Johnny cannot button his shirt, copy a square, dress himself or recognize colors. The Pediatrician concludes Johnny is functioning at the three year level, though he is five years of age (as a reader of *MIS*/KIDDING, you would arrive at the same estimate of developmental age by consulting Appendix I).

The Pediatrician suggests Johnny be tested by a Psychologist. Since Johnny's Mom cannot afford testing by a private psychologist, she requests her son's school to do the testing by the School Psychologist.

The results of IQ, Achievement and Social Maturity testing reveal that Johnny is Mildly Intellectually Limited (Mildly Mentally Retarded) and that his achievement levels are consistent with his ability levels; that is, Johnny's actual level of performance of academic tasks is at the level of his measured ability (his "IQ"). However, Johnny's Social Maturity tests are consistent with a diagnosis of Autism. In observing Johnny perform both in his mother's presence and in her absence, the School Psychologist concludes that Johnny also suffers from a high degree of anxiety whenever he is exposed to any change in routine or in the absence of his mother. Johnny often becomes completely incapacitated under these circumstances, making schooling very difficult. Johnny is referred to a Child Psychiatrist at a local health clinic.

The Child Psychiatrist sees Johnny several times in consultation with his mother, confirming the School Psychologist's findings. Since Johnny is able to perform at his level of ability only when anxiety is controlled, the Psychiatrist suggests enrolling Johnny in a small Special Education Class at the school, with a focus on developing social skills. To facilitate Johnny's engagement in the process, an anti-anxiety medication is prescribed and closely monitored.

Back at the school, an Individualized Educational Program (I.E.P.) is developed and Johnny begins the process of habilitation. Periodically, the Special Education teacher relays summaries of Johnny's progress to Mom who shares those observations with the prescribing Child Psychiatrist.

Can Kids With ASD's Grow Into Independently Functioning Adults?

The ultimate level of independence kids with ASD's can reach depends on their level of achievement of Activities of Daily Living. These activities include Basic abilities (self-care) and more advanced Instrumental abilities (necessary to live within a community):[6]

Basic ADL's

Basic ADL's consist of self-care tasks, including: 5

• Personal hygiene and grooming

• Dressing and undressing

• Feeding oneself

• Voluntarily controlling urine and bowel functions

• Ambulation

Instrumental ADL's

Instrumental ADL's are not basic, but allow independent living in a community:

• Housework

• Meal Preparation

• Taking medications

• Managing money

• Shopping for groceries or clothing

• Telephone use

• Using technology (as applicable)

- Adapted from Wikipedia: The Free Encyclopedia

For a wonderful fictional example of an adult with "functional" Asperger Disorder (note: NOT "disability!"), tune in to "The Big Bang Theory", a popular TV program in which the lead character, Sheldon, portrays the essential features of the Disorder, while "functioning" independently as a physicist. Though the program is comedic, it underscores the fact that high-functioning Autistic individuals can lead independent lives, though they may be considered "odd" in their mannerisms.

References:

1. DSM-IV-TR, American Psychiatric Association

2. Kanner L. Eisenberg, L Early Infantile Autism 1943-55, Am J Ortho- psychiatry 1956; 26:55-65

3. Wing L BMJ, Autistic Spectrum Disorders 1996;312:327-328

4. Wetherby A. Woods, J. Allen, L. Cleary, J. Dickinson, H. Lord, C. Early indicators of autism spectrum disorders in the second year of life. Journal of Autism and Developmental Disorders 2004: 34, 473-493.

5. McDowell, I., and Newell, C. 1996, Measuring Health: A Guide to Rating Scales and Questionnaires, 2nd edition. New York: Oxford University Press

6. Bookman, A., Harrington, M., Pass, L., & Reisner, E. 2007 - Family Caregiver Handbook. Cambridge, MA: Massachusetts Institute of Technology

CHAPTER NINE

Bipolar Disorder

What Is Bipolar Disorder (BPD)?

Bipolar Disorder is a form of IN/kidding characterized by:

- •Irritability (often mistaken for ADHD because it may include hyperactivity, recklessness [suggesting the "impulsivity" of ADHD] and distractibility.

- •Wide swings of emotion ("mood cycling"), ranging from depression (with associated withdrawal from usual activities, isolation, eating disturbances and suicidal thinking or acts) through unprovoked and violent episodes of rage (often resulting in physical harm to self or others) to "super" well being, including delusions of God-like powers.

- •Sleep disturbances, either too much sleep or too little.

- •A disconnect between antecedents and consequences. This means that kids with untreated BPD can't see how their acts ("antecedents") relate to the resulting bad things that happen to them ("consequences"). Or, to put it simply, they blame everyone else for what happens to them as a result of their *mis*/kidding. Typically, kids with untreated BPD have no remorse for their acts. It often appears as if their conscience has been obliterated.

The "hyperactive" components of BPD are referred to as "mania" and they may alternate with depressive symptoms. This is why BPD is sometimes referred to as "Manic-Depression." Not all kids with BPD exhibit all the symptoms mentioned and some may have mild enough symptoms that they fail to reach the "D" (Disorder) level of BPD. Seen through the *MIS*/KIDDING lens, a BP "tendency" (sometimes called "Cyclothymia") becomes Bipolar Disorder when the *mis*/kidding it causes reaches the *Mid*/kidding level; that is, when it accumulates more than 2 points on the *mis*/kidding thermometer. However, you've learned that scores of 1 or 2 on the *MIS*/KIDDING scale (that is, *mini*/kidding) are not worthy of your efforts at intervention. So it's possible to have Cyclothymia that never reaches a *Mid*/kidding or higher level. While you'd be aware of a certain level of moodiness, irritability or bad choice-making, the minimal impact of the *mis*/kidding on the Consequence Areas of Age Work, Others or Authority, not (yet) having reached the *Mid*/kidding level, would allow you to ignore its unpleasantness until or unless it escalated to a higher level.

What Causes BPD?

BPD is thought to be caused by a disturbance in brain chemicals ("neurotransmitters") within the emotion centers of the brain. These disturbances are often inherited from one generation to another, though "new" cases do occur without a known affected relative. It's been reported that between 40 – 70% of identical twins and 5 – 10% of first degree relatives (parents, brothers/sisters, offspring of an affected parent) will share a diagnosis of BPD.[1]

Because BPD causes great suffering, not only for those close to the affected person and those targeted by the *mis*/kidding, but for the affected individual, it is not uncommon for older kids with BPD to attempt to "self-medicate" with alcohol and other drugs. As one kid said, "Do you think it's fun being mad all the time?" Another said, "I wish I could want to live, like other kids!"

Though substance abuse does not cause BPD, it plays upon the abnormal chemistry of BPD, intensifying the symptoms and often elevating them to the level of *KILLER*/kidding.

Of greatest importance is the fact that BPD is *not* a *willful* condition. That is, kids can't decide not to have BPD. BPD takes away kids' choice-making and, until it is treated, discipline, including rewards and punishments, will not solve the *mis*/kidding.

Its Beginnings

BPD in all its forms may affect as many as 1-2 adults in a hundred over a lifetime.[2] The symptoms may appear suddenly and without warning, or emerge slowly over years and eventually intensify to a diagnostic level.

In severe cases, especially when close relatives on both sides of the family have been diagnosed with BPD, the condition can be suspected by Behavioral-Developmental Pediatricians and Child Psychiatrists even by three years of age. Because BPD is a life-long condition and its formal recognition may seriously limit entry into certain careers, a definitive diagnosis is usually deferred until typical treatment for BPD has been effective and required for several years.

BPD in kids most typically emerges with the approach of adolescence, though as noted above, the rudiments of the condition may be seen much earlier.

Does BPD Occur With Other Conditions?

Physicians know, "You can have as many diseases as you pleases." In the case of BPD, it is very common for other forms of *mis*/kidding to "co-occur." Among the most common co-occurring conditions in kids are ADHD, Autistic Spectrum Disorders, Developmental Delay, Epilepsy and, in older kids, substance abuse. Because BPD represents an abnormality of brain chemistry rendering a kid more vulnerable to stress, child abuse in any form may elevate a BP "tendency" to overt BPD – often to the level of *KILLER*/kidding.

What Are The Consequences of Untreated BPD?

The irritability of BPD can easily be mistaken for ADHD, since it may be associated with inattentiveness, hyperactivity and impulsivity (doing things without thinking about consequences). If the irritability of BPD is mistaken for ADHD and treated with stimulant medications (like methylphenidate or amphetamines), the emotion centers of the brain may be "stimulated" causing worsening of the mood cycling of BPD and driving the *mis*/kidding to the *KILLER*/kidding level.

Wide swings of mood, or "mood cycling, may reach suicidal depths of depression, while anger episodes may reach levels of rage that result in destructive acts, harm to others or even homicide. Manic episodes can result in recklessness, resulting in lawlessness, injury or even death.

Sleep disturbances in kids may affect overall health, including weight loss, weight gain, falling grades, menstrual problems and heightened depression or anger.

Most dangerous of all is the disconnect between antecedents and consequences. This is the essence of In/kidding. Kids with untreated BPD will regularly meet the criteria for *mis*/kidding by assaulting the Consequence Areas. They cannot achieve consistently in the *physical, social* and *communication* areas of Age Work, relate normally to Others or submit to reasonable Authority (follow rules).

Can Bipolar Disorder Be Treated Without Medication?

The In/kidding of BPD means that persuasion, motivation, rewards and punishments will fail to resolve the *mis*/kidding until or unless the brain is able to "cool" irritability, diminish mood cycling and "reconnect" antecedents and consequences with effective treatment. While it is true that kids suffering from untreated BPD may, to some extent, learn to defuse "triggering events" that lead to depression, anger and recklessness, thus reserving a place for counseling and therapy in the treatment strategy, these interventions cannot succeed on their own over the long term until brain function is restored.

Effective treatment for BPD requires the assistance of medical professionals, including the use of medication to restore abnormal brain chemistry.

What Medicines Are Used To Treat BPD and How Do They Work?

The symptoms of BPD vary from one kid to another. Though each of the components of BPD are usually present to some extent in any kid with BPD, only those components reaching a level of *Mid*/kidding at any given time require treatment. Since several components of BPD almost always coexist, several medications must often be prescribed together to achieve control. This "polypharmacy" is a frequent and necessary occurrence in the treatment of BPD.

Here follows a list of some commonly prescribed medications along with targeted BPD components. The list is necessarily incomplete because new agents are being introduced constantly in an attempt to increase effectiveness and decrease side effects:

Irritability and Wide Swings of Mood (Including Mania & Depression):

Anticonvulsants	Antipsychotics	Antidepressants
• Oxcarbazepine	• Risperdone	• Fluoxetine
• Lamotrigine	• Haloperidol	• Sertaline
• Divalproex	• Lithium	• Citalopram
• Topiramate	• Quetiapine	• Paroxetine
• Carbamazepine	• Aripiprazole	• Escitalopram
	• Ziprasidone	• Bupropion

The anticonvulsants work by toning down the excitability of emotion-controlling brain cells. They may, unfortunately, also sedate other parts of the brain and, in some cases, cause more serious side effects, like suppressing white blood cells or irritating the liver.

The antidepressants affect the interaction of brain chemicals (neurotransmitters) with nerve cells in the emotion centers of the brain. Because these medications not only elevate mood (overcome depression), but also decrease anxiety, they may at times reduce anxiety too much, resulting in recklessness. Among the most dangerous of potential side effects is the reduction of anxiety to the point of enabling suicidal thinking to progress to suicidal acts. The dosing of antidepressants requires a careful balance between elevating mood and avoiding recklessness.

The antipsychotics also affect the workings of neurotransmitters in the brain. This group of medications has potentially serious side effects, including effects on metabolism and muscle function. Usually, the effects of these medications on the body are monitored with periodic blood tests.

As is always the case, a decision to use any of the medications must weigh the risks of using the medication against the need to control the potentially life-altering or life-threatening *mis*/kidding of BPD.

Sleep Disturbances:

Sleep-Inducing Antidepressants

- Mirtazapine
- Trazodone

Other "Sedating" Medications

- Estazolam
- Diphenhydramine
- Flurazepam
- Clonidine

Medications used to promote sleep in kids with BPD cover a wide range of categories. Side effects vary, but in general, care must be taken to avoid dependency or addiction, a significant risk with benzodiazepines such as Estazolam and Flurazepam listed above.

The "Disconnect" Between Antecedents and Consequences

Arguably, the most serious aspect of BPD is the loss of kids' ability to intuitively comprehend the consequences of their acts. When the intensity of emotions, heightened by mood cycling, provokes suicidal thinking, rage or a feeling of God-like power, kids may engage in *KILLER*/kidding without any recognition its significance or consequences for themselves or others. To them, such acts are a "normal" and reasonable response to the world and any of its inhabitants. This is the true meaning of the term "psychotic", and psychotic or "crazy" kidding is potentially the most dangerous of BPD's attributes.

Over the years, several generations of "antipsychotic" medications have been developed. Some of the more commonly prescribed antipsychotics have been listed above. The biochemistry of the effects of these medications on the psychotic thinking of BPD and other related conditions is beyond the scope of this book. Suffice it to say that both the definitive diagnosis and treatment of BPD in a kid will require the scrutiny of a Child Psychiatrist. However, the recognition and categorization of the *mis*/kidding of BPD is well within the capabilities of anyone familiar with the *Mis*/kidding process.

Who's Responsible For Recognizing BPD?

BPD can first be recognized as a problem worth doing something about when it results in *Mid*/kidding (or worse). Though the *mis*/kidding may not be recognized as BPD at this stage, or conversely, may be suspected of being BPD while actually being another "masquerading" condition (such as Cyclothymia, hyperthyroidism, lead poisoning, ADHD, etc), its identification as *mis*/kidding, its classification as *Mid*/kidding (or even *KILLER*/kidding) and its characterization as In/kidding can be achieved by anyone familiar with the *Mis*/kidding Process as outlined in the previous chapters of this book. This includes professionals, parents or even kids themselves.

Once we recognize In/kidding at the *Mid*/kidding level, we know that professional assistance must be sought for definitive diagnosis and treatment, in the following order:

Physician (1°Care &/ or Child Neurologist) ⟶ *Psychiatrist* ⟶ *Educator*

What 1° Care Physicians (Pediatricians) And Neurologists Do For Kids With BPD

Pediatricians and Neurologists begin by reviewing the family's history of medical conditions to identify risks. They must rule out any process that might cause ongoing damage, such as brain degeneration, lead poisoning, an overactive thyroid gland or a seizure disorder. Medicines taken for other reasons may contribute to or even cause BPD-like symptoms. For example, stimulant medications prescribed for ADHD can intensify emotion in kids with Cyclothymia and other Mood Disorders, elevating them to levels suggestive of BPD.

Associated neurological conditions, like Tourette Disorder, Cerebral Palsy, Autistic Spectrum Disorders, Epilepsy or brain tumors need to be identified and treated.

The doctor may next gather observations from teachers and family members to compare kids' behaviors in different settings. This should confirm the "non-selective" nature of the In/kidding (that is, it occurs everywhere) and may help distinguish different forms of BPD.

Physical and neurological examinations usually follow. Laboratory tests, including blood work, an EEG or even an MRI brain scan may be ordered. It is at this point that conditions masquerading as BPD or complicating its presence will be recognized.

After the *physical* component of Age Work has been assessed by the Pediatrician or Child Neurologist, threats to the *social* component of Age Work need to be evaluated by a Child Psychiatrist.

What Child Psychiatrists Do For BPD

Child Psychiatrists are familiar with the many mental illnesses that cause irritability, mood cycling, sleep disorders and psychotic ("crazy") *mis*/kidding in kids. They routinely investigate a family's history of mental illness, the evolution of a kid's symptoms, the degree of danger threatening the kid and others and the co-occurrence of substance abuse. They are able to distinguish BPD from other mental health conditions and recognize different forms of BPD. These determinations allow the Child Psychiatrist to construct a treatment strategy, usually employing both medication to restore brain function and counseling and therapy to confer on the kid a degree of control over *mis*/kidding.

What Educators Do For BPD

Because classroom teachers spend so much time with kids, their ongoing observations are extremely valuable and provide the managing Child Psychiatrist a "set of eyes" to adjust both medications and the focus of counseling or therapy.

School Counselors and School Psychologists can provide "free", on-site interventions for episodic *mis*/kidding.

The irritability of BPD may depress classroom performance and its psychotic components may affect rule-following and interpersonal relationships. By communicating such ongoing observations to the Child Psychiatrist, Educators contribute immeasurably to the effective treatment of BPD.

When Can We Stop Treating BPD?

BPD is a "forever" condition. Because sudden stressors like the death of a loved one, parental separation or divorce, bullying or physical illness may trigger BPD symptoms that reach the *Mid*/kidding level and thus require intervention, the easing or removal of stress may "cool" the level of *mis*/kidding to *mini*/kidding and intermittently obviate the need for treatment. Nevertheless, a kid's vulnerability to recurrence of BPD symptoms remains. Keeping in mind the fact that the psychotic symptoms of BPD are not usually recognized by an affected kid when they occur, it is critical for such kids to be monitored by someone they can trust so that recurrent symptoms are recognized early and effective treatment is provided.

Many kids, when they feel "normal" and are achieving satisfactorily in school "on" medication, will stop taking their meds. When the symptoms of BPD recur, these kids may continue to feel "normal" as their *mis*/kidding climbs in intensity, once again reaching the level of *Mid*/kidding or even *KILLER*/kidding.

References:

1. Craddock N, Jones I, J. Med. Genetics, 1999 36:585-594

2. Correll C, Hauser MA, Medscape Psychiatry & Mental Health, Posted 1/04/2011

CHAPTER TEN

Cerebral Palsy

What Is Cerebral Palsy?

Cerebral palsy is a nervous system condition caused by damage to the brain and spinal cord early in life and primarily affecting the *physical* component of Age Work; specifically, movement, posture and coordination. The nervous system injury doesn't progress, though associated impairments may lead to greater disability as time goes on.

Its Beginnings

Injuries that cause cerebral palsy always occur during the early developmental period; that is, while kids' brains are rapidly physically maturing – usually in the uterus (before birth), immediately after birth or during the first few months of life. Impairments affecting brain function after the early developmental period, like strokes or auto accidents and any events or conditions that incur ongoing injury, like brain tumors and PKU, though each may result in brain damage and a seizure disorder, do not qualify as "cerebral palsy."

How Does Cerebral Palsy Create Mis/kidding?

Cerebral palsy occurs in all degrees of severity and is usually accompanied by damage to other areas of the nervous system that control functions beyond movement, posture and coordination. Because injuries that cause "CP" are rarely limited to areas of the brain that control muscle function, learning, attentiveness, emotionality and overall intelligence can all be affected.

The innate limitations imposed on kids by CP, such as weakness, stiffness, spasticity or writhing movements, create In/kidding. Kids act "strangely" and provoke those around them to react with annoyance, Confusion, Anxiety or FEAR, the emotional "yardsticks" of *mis*/kidding. Frustrated by the constraints of their condition, affected kids may react to the

169

perceptions of others by acting out, thus adding Out/kidding to the In/kidding of CP.

Mis/kidding occurs when CP adversely affects any of the Consequence Areas (Age Work, Others, Authority). The severity of the *mis*/kidding is determined by the "degrees" generated on the *Mis*/kidding Scale. CP may lead to *mini*/kidding, like the "klutzy" kid, which can be ignored, *Mid*/kidding, which if ignored will eventually become threatening and for which a strategy must be developed, or *KILLER*/kidding, which may kill a kid or others and which demands immediate and forceful intervention.

How Does CP Affect Age Work?

Though CP always impacts the *physical* component of Age Work, physical impairments, in turn, may threaten *social* skills and the physical *communication* of intelligence. Thus Age Work in its entirety may be delayed. Such delays in Age Work are easily recognized by most parents, usually (but not always) within the first year of life. However, subtle forms of CP, first encountered as delayed Age Work, may not be recognized as CP until or unless professional assessment and diagnosis is sought.

How Can CP Threaten The Social Component of Age Work?

CP traps kids in bodies that don't do what they want them to do. The more intelligent kids are the more frustrating CP is for them. Unintelligible or misarticulated speech patterns may affect interpersonal relationships by early elementary school years. Frustration may lead to aggression or withdrawal, eventually reaching the level of *Mid*/kidding or even *KILLER*/kidding. Peers, teachers and even parents, unaware of underlying CP, may not recognize this form of In/kidding and misinterpret it as willful opposition. Attempts to coerce compliance may worsen the *social* component of Age Work.

How Can CP Impair The Communication Component Of Age Work?

The *communication* component of Age Work includes both the verbal and non-verbal interchange of thoughts. This includes speech, physical demeanor (through which much emotion is conveyed) and motoric skills, like writing, drawing and gesturing. Impaired *physical* skills may thus threaten all aspects of *communication* ability. In severe cases, there may be no way to adequately assess intelligence.

What Causes CP?

CP can be caused by any injurious event affecting the growth or maturation of the brain and spinal cord during the early developmental period. Damage or destruction of fetus' or infants' developing nerve cells can be caused, for example, by alcohol or other drug use during pregnancy, malnutrition and even prescribed medications used during pregnancy and can result in CP. For these reasons and many others, prenatal care under the aegis of a well-trained professional is highly recommended.

During labor and delivery, a precise sequence of biologically "programmed" steps takes place to transform babies from aquatic to air breathing creatures. If these steps fail to provide adequate circulation, temperature regulation, essential nutrients and oxygenation, damage will occur to the central nervous system and may result in CP. During the birth process, some infants, especially premature babies, may bleed into the brain. This is a common cause of CP in such infants.

For several weeks after birth, infant brains and spinal cords are very susceptible to damage from infections, high fever, toxins and fluctuating levels of blood chemicals. Meningitis, strep infections, low blood sugar and high levels of yellow jaundice in babies are all potential causes of CP.

How Common Is CP & Who's Most At Risk?

CP is estimated to occur in about one to three of every thousand live births. It's much more common in premature babies, especially those with very low birth weights. It's also more common in twins, triplets and higher multiple births. Because couples with infertility are being helped to get pregnant with techniques and medicines that increase the likelihood of multiple births, the occurrence of CP within this group is also more common. CP is also more common in babies born to mothers over forty years of age.

Though medical technology has increasingly protected most "big" babies from CP, it saves tinier and more premature infants among whom CP is more likely. Further, by allowing older couples to become pregnant, the risk of CP increases for these infants. Thus, in spite of major medical advances, the incidence of CP has remained remarkably consistent over the years.

What Are The Symptoms Of Cerebral Palsy?

CP impairs normal movement and posture. Brain and spinal cord nerve cells, damaged or destroyed during early life, can't fully control muscle movements in various parts of the body. Since muscles need nerve cells to function properly and to remain healthy, muscles that are connected to damaged nerve cells become damaged in turn. In CP, muscles may display "paresis" or "hypotonia" (forms of weakness), "hypertonia" or "spasticity" (forms of tightness), "dystonia" (abnormal load-bearing or "springiness"), or combinations of these disorders. "Choreoathetosis" and "ballismus" (abnormal movements) may also be seen.

CP always affects muscle control, but depending upon which other areas of the central nervous system are damaged, additional impairments may equal or exceed the impact of the muscle-control problems. Developmental and Learning Disabilities, AD(H)D, Epilepsy, speech impediments, body deformities, poor or absent bowel or bladder control, deafness or blindness and Mental Retardation commonly coexist with CP.

The impairments associated with CP may be so mild as to be unnoticeable to all but the trained eye, or so severe as to cause total immobility and isolation.

How Early In Life Can Cerebral Palsy Be Diagnosed?

CP can be suspected in the newborn nursery when a baby suffers damage to the brain or spinal cord. However, except in the most severe cases, the diagnosis of CP requires the passage of time because babies are able to compensate for damage in one area of the brain by using undamaged areas. What appears to be a serious movement or postural disorder in the nursery may improve later.

In general, delays in muscle control and abnormal reflexes of various types allow Developmental Pediatricians and Child Neurologists to diagnose CP in the majority of moderate to severely affected kids by one year of age. Mildly affected kids rarely benefit from early diagnosis and may be mislabeled if diagnosed before two or three years of age.

Cerebral Palsy Can Only Be Diagnosed When It Causes Mis/kidding

There's no single symptom or sign that's specific for CP. Likewise, there's no single test that can be used to diagnose CP. The condition is suspected whenever 1) damage to the central nervous system is accompanied by 2) abnormal muscle control. These two observations of central nervous system damage and abnormal muscle control can be made by anyone who spends time with kids, such as family members, babysitters, teachers, psychologists or doctors. Indeed, most cases of CP are first suspected by non-physicians.

Damage to the nervous system and abnormal muscle control are only recognizable by their effects on the Consequence Areas. Thus CP and all the conditions that masquerade as CP first proclaim themselves as *mis*/kidding. This means you don't have to be a professional to recognize the need for diagnosis or to manage the steps in achieving the diagnosis. All you need to do is to apply the *Mis*/kidding Process.

Getting Proper Diagnosis & Treatment For Cerebral Palsy

If you're a parent, the *Mis*/kidding Process provides an outline for action. It prompts you to start with an assessment of physical conditions that may be causing impairments over which your kid may have no volitional control. This is achieved by seeking a physician's medical examination. It next reminds you to proceed with psychological assessment of potential disabilities imposed by those physical impairments. It then guides you to seek educational assessment and intervention for disabilities or handicaps.

Here are the steps taken in the diagnostic phase of the *Mis*/kidding Process when you suspect CP:

First step;

To recognize *mis*/kidding, check the Consequence Areas-

Age Work: Is there a threat to *physical* development, such as abnormal muscle control? Are social skills threatened? Are *communication* skills delayed?

Others: Are there threats to or complaints from Others, including yourself?

Authority: Does the kidding threaten Authority?

If the answer to any of these questions is "yes", you've identified *mis*/kidding and you need to go on to Step Two. If none of the Consequence Areas are affected, you can stop here.

Second step;

Distinguish *KILLER*/KIDDING and *Mid*/kidding from *mini*/kidding-

1.Check your emotional reaction to the *mis*/kidding and assign "degrees":

"cool"(annoyance)	= 1 degree
"Warm"(Anxiety, Anger, Confusion)	= 2 degrees
"HOT"(FEAR)	= 3 degrees

2.Check effects on Consequence Areas and assign "degrees":

Age Work……………………… ……	up to 3 degrees
-*physical*	= 1 degree

-*social*	= 1 degree
-*communication*	= 1 degree
Others....................	Up to 2 degrees
-You	= 1 degree
-Everyone else	= 1 degree
Authority...............	= 1 degree

3. Add the total "degrees" to define the intensity of the *Mis*/kidding:

KILLER/kidding	= 7, 8, or 9 degrees
Mid/kidding	= 3, 4, 5, or 6 degrees
mini/kidding	= 1 or 2 degrees

If you've discovered *mini*/kidding, you can stop here and ignore it. If you've discovered *KILLER*/kidding, "cool" it to *Mid*/kidding immediately if you can, or get help. If you suspect In/kidding at either the *KILLER*/kidding or *Mid*/kidding level and need help to diagnose or manage it, proceed to the next step:

Third step:

Isolate In/kidding. It affects Age Work and-

-"_looks_"-	and	"_feels_"-	_Degrees_ =	_Intensity_
		annoying	(1-2)	mini/kidding
-non-selective		Confusing		
-unpredictable		or	(3-6)	Mid/kidding
-of no benefit		Anxiety-provoking		
		FEAR-provoking	(7-9)	KILLER/kidding

Choose a professional helper for each affected skill area of Age Work as follows:

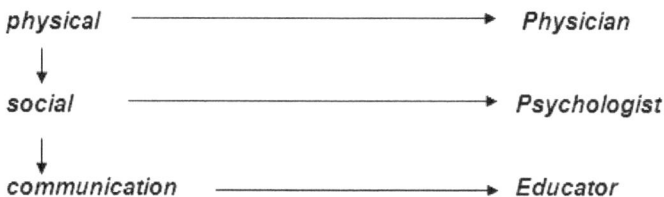

physical ⟶ *Physician*

↓

social ⟶ *Psychologist*

↓

communication ⟶ *Educator*

If you suspect CP and have identified In/kidding, a physician experienced in the diagnosis of brain and spinal cord conditions, such as a Developmental Pediatrician or a Child Neurologist, should perform a complete medical examination. This is a critical step because some conditions that look like CP aren't CP. They can cause progressive damage or even kill a kid. Remember, the nervous system damage in CP does not worsen over time. It's absolutely imperative to be sure the condition really is CP so that the expectation of progress from that time forth rests on a solid base.

What Physicians Do For CP

Physicians who are knowledgeable about CP can't provide all the medical treatments CP kids need, especially if impairments are moderate or severe. But they can coordinate the efforts of a team of specialists. Because of the complexity of treating multiple impairments, a parent must insist on designating a medical specialist who will be their kid's case manager. This is a person the family can turn to for information and advice and who can help to decide when and if more or less intervention is advisable. Here's a list of some medical specialists who help kids with CP:

- Developmental Pediatricians act as case managers.

- Child Neurologists treat complex nervous system disorders.

- Orthopedists help with bone and joint problems.

- Physiotherapists help manage physical disorders of CP.

- Occupational Therapists help develop self-help skills.

- Biomedical Engineers design equipment to enhance mobility and communication.

- Neurosurgeons operate to improve nervous system function.

What Do Psychologists Do For CP?

Psychologists measure peoples' capabilities, achievements and social functioning. Before two and a half to three years of age, psychological tests rely on what kids do rather than what they say; that is, they rely on kids' muscle activities (sitting, standing, walking, toileting, drawing, dressing, playing) to determine developmental maturity. After about three years of age as maturation continues, "normal" kids use language well enough that *communication* skills become an ever greater component of measured "intelligence."

Though muscle-control and language skills are parts of "intelligence", muscle-control is the least important and also the least reliable component of intelligence. It is, of course, the central disorder of CP and renders the measurement of "intelligence" in CP a major challenge.

When the usual IQ tests are applied to kids with moderate or severe CP they often appear retarded. That's because their bodies are unable to perform required muscle-dependent skills. Even when mental retardation is present, these kids appear more retarded than they really are (or will be when they are older). The younger the CP kid when tested with standard measures, the more dismal the apparent IQ.

After the physical disorders of CP have been identified by the medical team, the degree of "disability" they're causing needs to be measured accurately. The best equipped professional to perform these measures is the Clinical Child Psychologist. Keeping in mind that tests given to young kids with CP always show less ability than will be seen at older ages, this baseline provides a "starting point" for periodic comparison with additional tests as interventions proceed. The baseline allows progress to be tracked over time. Since kids with CP always improve in ability over time, failure to do so as interventions are tracked mean that they either have something more than CP or they're not getting the help they need.

Clinical Child Psychologists provide at least two critical services; they measure baseline abilities and they objectively track progress. They are also able to work with the anger and frustration experienced by kids with CP. Families need to be counseled about their kids' capabilities and advised how to engage them in social situations without creating more anger and frustration. Overprotecting kids with CP may feel good at first for both parents and kids, but kids' self esteem rests not only on parental love, but on honest achievement. To develop self esteem, the ultimate basis for independence, kids sometimes need to be "pushed" in spite of their impairments. Clinical Child Psychologists can advise when and how to apply the "push."

What Do Educators Do For Kids With CP?

CP becomes a handicapping condition only when it prevents kids from engaging in "life, liberty and the pursuit of happiness" up to their level of ability. CP kids need to be able to communicate their desires and capabilities to loved ones and to their communities. Teaching kids how to use their physical and intellectual strengths and avoid being "disabled" by CP is best accomplished by Educators. The bewildering array of titles Educators use to describe themselves, many of which have been presented in Chapter

Three of Part I, attest to the myriad of paths kids may travel to overcome disability:

- Speech and Language Clinicians and Speech Pathologists help kids overcome learning differences and unintelligible speech.

- Learning Disability and Special Education Teachers help kids to acquire, utilize and express knowledge with techniques that compensate for learning differences and deficits.

- Perceptual Motor Specialists help kids use their bodies to communicate desires, and acquire and demonstrate skills.

- Service Coordinators (from local county agencies) construct and implement Individualized Family Service Plans (IFSP's) for kids from birth to 3 yrs of age.

- School Psychologists track kids' academic and emotional progress and help design Individualized Educational Programs (IEP's) for kids 3yrs of age and older.

- Pupil Personnel Workers assess strengths and vulnerabilities of kids and their families, helping them adjust to disabilities and assisting in finding and utilizing community support services.

Because Educators spend more time observing and working with kids than any other professionals, they can provide ongoing surveillance of kids' progress, identifying benefits and shortcomings of other professionals' interventions. Wise and experienced Physicians and Psychologists (as well as parents) caring for kids with CP monitor Educators' in-school observations closely and revise their treatment plans accordingly.

Remember The Difference Between "Disorder" and "Disability!

The key to reducing the "disability" of CP to a mere "disorder" is to enable a kid with CP to achieve levels of performance consistent with ability. For this to happen, a CP kid's abilities must be assessed at least yearly, since they will appear to change continually, often for the better.

Medical diagnosis, psychological evaluation and educational interventions are the basis for ongoing progress.

When speech, writing or typing or even sign language are beyond the physical capabilities of a CP kid, new technologies can be used to enable communication. Biomedical engineers continue to design mechanical and electronic systems for virtually any physical impairment. These "artificial" systems allow such kids to "escape" the confines of CP by communicating more readily. Community resources, often identified by Pupil Personnel (or Social) Workers, are available to help fund these interventions.

The motor impairments of CP are one condition that kids CAN occasionally outgrow. That's why it's important NOT to base predictions or expectations on the results of initial tests.

CHAPTER ELEVEN

Developmental Delay and Mental Retardation

What Is Developmental Delay?

Developmental delay is an umbrella term used to describe the failure of kids to acquire anticipated skills at the right times during the early years of life. The phrase covers any and all delays during the "developmental period", including, but not limited to, intellectual delay. Viewed through the *Mis*/kidding Process, Developmental Delay is present when a kid displays significant delay in any skill area(s) of Age Work (*physical, social, communication*) reaching the *Mid*/kidding or higher level.

What's The Difference Between Developmental Delay & Mental Retardation

Mental retardation is a more specific term than developmental delay, and is deferred until a kid reaches at least 3 yrs of age or older (when IQ measures become more reliable). The diagnosis requires psychological testing with evidence of an IQ less than 70, impairment in at least 2 areas of "adaptive behavior" and recognition of the condition before adulthood (usually by 18 years of age). Viewed through the *Mis*/kidding Process, Mental Retardation is recognized by a kid's consistent delays in the *social* and *communication* areas of Age Work, during the developmental period (before adulthood), reaching the *Mid*/kidding or higher level.

What Is The "Developmental Period" & Why Is It Important?

The developmental period is that time in life when events occurring outside kids' brains, though sometimes located in other parts of their bodies, directly influence the physical construction and connectivity of their brains. This malleability or "plasticity" of kids' brains during early development makes them peculiarly susceptible to destructive processes that act on the brain at this time, often creating life-long impairments.

Here are some examples of destructive processes occurring during the developmental period that can cause long-term impairments:

- •Kids deprived of love and affection, though well fed, may fail to grow normally.

- •Kids suffering frequent or persistent ear infections can develop speech or language disabilities.

- •Kids who are "cross-eyed" during the first 3 yrs of life may develop amblyopia, or partial blindness, which persists even after the eye deviation is corrected.

The possibility that kids' brains are "plastic" enough to respond to early intervention, and that their performance may eventually catch up, injects a note of optimism into the phrase "developmental delay." Conversely, the phrase "mental retardation" suggests that brain processes are irrevocably delayed and will remain so for life.

Just as destructive processes can act on the immature brain to create chronic disabilities, early identification and intervention for developmental delay offer opportunities to utilize brain plasticity to promote compensatory brain function with catch up in performance.

Here are some examples of the compensatory effects of early identification and intervention for developmental delay:

- •Babies who can't see well, but whose visual impairments are identified and corrected early in life do better in reading and visual-motor skills than similar kids whose vision is corrected later in life.

- •Kids with hearing impairments who are identified in infancy and whose hearing is boosted with hearing aids develop more advanced language skills than those whose hearing is corrected later or not at all.

- •Kids with delayed school readiness who are enrolled in educational enrichment programs, such as Head Start, perform at higher academic levels than similar kids without intervention for at least several years after leaving the program.

The "Developmental Period" Ends Sometime In Elementary School

There's no precise end to the developmental period. One reason is that different kids' brains develop at different rates within a wide "normal" range. Kids may progress rapidly within a skill area one year and slowly within the same skill area another year. One kid's pattern of development may be different from that of another, yet both may be normal.

The developmental period, characterized by the brain's ability to adjust to and even compensate for environmental influences and heredity, winds down in the elementary school years, though a degree of brain "plasticity" persists into adult life. Were this not so, physical and occupational therapy for adult stroke victims and those suffering from other brain injuries as adults wouldn't result in long-term improvement, yet they do.

Professionals study "normal" development and attempt to diagnose causes of developmental delay by testing streams of development. Each stream of development depends on many contributory body processes, most of which can't be accurately measured in preschoolers. Developmental tests experts use to measure streams of development give way to more precise tests as kids enter the elementary school years. Specific diagnoses begin to emerge at that time to explain delays. By the middle to the end of the elementary school years, most medical diagnoses have been made and those kids destined to "catch up" have done so. At that point, the term "developmental delay" loses its meaning along with its optimistic connotation and specific, persistent disabilities or mental retardation must be suspected.

Delayed Developmental Streams Are Recognized As Mis/kidding

Skills that result from the interaction of environment and brain capabilities during the developmental period are described by researchers in terms of five "developmental streams":

- Language: Receiving, comprehending and expressing thoughts and desires.

- Visual-motor: Eye-hand coordination. A measure of non-verbal problem solving.

- Gross motor: Body control.

- Social: Interpersonal relationships with others.

- Activities of daily living: Measures of self-sufficiency and independence.

These "streams" are the basis of developmental testing and each has critical "markers" at various ages to define the limits of "normal" versus "delay." Delays within any stream guide professionals to perform specific tests for accurate diagnosis. Parents and caretakers can simplify the recognition of developmental delay and manage evaluations and interventions by "bundling" these streams of normal development into the three skill areas of Age Work: *physical, social* and *communication*:

- •*physical* skills include control of large and small muscles, including eye-hand coordination.

- •*social* skills encompass social adaptive abilities, including activities of daily living.

- •*communication* skills include academic performance and verbal and non-verbal language, both receptive and expressive, through which academic competence is displayed.

Using the *Mis*/kidding Process to recognize developmental delay by its threat to the skill areas of Age Work, any of the following conditions may emerge:

- • Mental Retardation will present as non-progressive delays in *social* and *communication* skill areas.

- • Cerebral Palsy will present with delays in *physical* and often *communication* skill areas.

- • AD(H)D may cause delays in *physical, social* and/or *communication* areas.

- • Blindness and deafness (partial or complete) will present with delays in *social* and *communication* areas.

- • Undiagnosed physical illness will present with delays in any or all skill areas of Age Work.

- • Mental illness including Bipolar Disorder and Depression will cause delays in *social* and *communication* areas.

- • Autistic Spectrum Disorders will present as delays in *social* and *communication* areas.

- • Substance abuse will present with delays in all areas of Age Work.

- • Learning disabilities will present with delays in *communication* areas.

To recognize developmental delay, we don't need to remember which streams of development flow into which skill areas of Age Work. We do need to remember that *mis*/kidding is defined by delay in any component of Age Work and that if it reaches a level of *Mid*/kidding or higher, intervention is necessary.

How to Get Proper Diagnosis & Treatment for Developmental Delay

Identifying a developmental delay is merely another way of saying you've encountered *mis*/kidding. It doesn't mean Mental Retardation is present. Both Out/kidding (kids' conscious or unconscious choice-making) and In/kidding (innate conditions that limit choice-making) can cause delay within any skill area of Age Work. Here are some examples:

Out/kidding causing developmental delay:

- •Kids who have never been offered the use of a cup during the first year of life, having been drinking only from a bottle, may refuse the cup at 15 months and so "fail" to achieve that "critical marker" of *social* development for that age.

- •Kids raised in a bilingual or trilingual family may articulate less than half their vocabulary intelligibly at three years of age and so miss "critical markers" in *communication* development for that age.

In/kidding causing developmental delay-

- •Kids with the physical impairments of cerebral palsy or partial blindness may show no interest in playing "pat-a-cake" at 10 months or imitating activities at 12 months, thus missing those "critical markers" of *physical and social* development for those ages.

- •Kids with Autistic Spectrum Disorders may not use personal pronouns, like "I" and "she", by 3 years of age, thus missing that "critical marker" of *communication* ability.

For these reasons, the three initial steps of the diagnostic phase of the *Mis*/kidding process need to be followed for every kid with developmental delay.

Leaving out even one step can be dangerous! Not only are parents likely to miss hidden conditions, but even professionals in one discipline can miss conditions familiar to those in other disciplines.

Here are the steps to take if you discover developmental delay:

First step:

Recognize *mis*/kidding by checking the Consequence Areas-

- **Age Work**: Are there any delays of "critical markers" in *physical, social* or *communication* skill areas? (See Appendix I).

- **Others**: Have Others, including yourself, complained of or been affected by the kidding?

- **Authority**: Is the kidding threatening Authority?

If the answer to any of these questions is "yes", you've identified *mis*/kidding and you need to go on to Step Two. If none of the Consequence Areas are affected, you can stop here.

<u>Second step:</u>

Distinguish *KILLER*/kidding and *Mid*/kidding from *mini*/kidding-

1. Check your emotional reaction to the *mis*/kidding and assign "degrees":

"cool"= annoyance   = 1 degree

"Warm"= Anxiety, Anger, Confusion   = 2 degrees

"HOT"=FEAR   = 3 degrees

2. Check effects on Consequence Areas and count "degrees":

- Age Work…………………………...Up to 3 degrees

 -physical   = 1

 -social   = 1

 -communication   = 1

- Others……………………………… Up to 2 degrees

 (You)   = 1

 (Everyone else)   = 1

- Authority…………………………… 1 degree

3. Add the "degrees" to define the intensity of the *mis*/kidding:

KILLER/kidding   = 7, 8, or 9 degrees

 Mid/kidding   = 3, 4, 5, or 6 degrees

 mini/kidding   = 1 or 2 degrees

If you've discovered only *mini*/kidding, you can stop here and ignore it. Kids who show isolated delays rather than patterns of delay don't require intervention at the mini/kidding level.

If you've identified *KILLER*/kidding, "cool" it to *Mid*/kidding immediately, if you can. If you need help or have discovered *Mid*/kidding, proceed to the next step.

Third step:

Isolate In/kidding. It affects Age Work and-

-"*looks*"-	and	"*feels*"-	Degrees	=	Intensity
		annoying	(1-2)		mini/kidding
-non-selective		Confusing			
-unpredictable		or	(3-6)		Mid/kidding
-of no benefit		Anxiety-provoking			
		FEAR-provoking	(7-9)		KILLER/kidding

After you've stopped *KILLER*/kidding and laid aside any *mini*/kidding, you've got time to investigate and manage *Mid*/kidding. If you've limited the *Mid*/kidding to Out/kidding (willful *mis*/kidding), you can proceed through Steps Four and Five, using the HoNoR Role to design and energize your own W/L Commands for good/kidding, or you can follow one or another of my favorite "recipes" in Appendix IV to do so.

If you suspect In/kidding or need expert help to stop *KILLER*/kidding, choose a professional for each affected skill area of Age Work in this order:

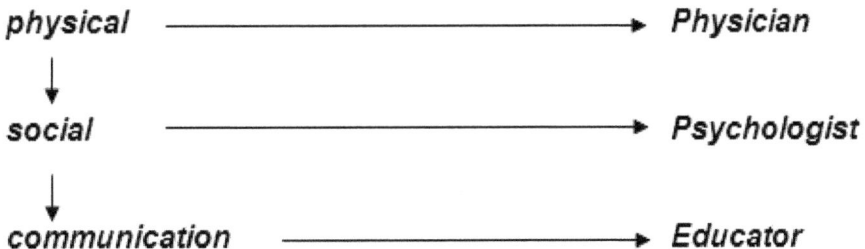

physical ⟶ **Physician**

↓

social ⟶ **Psychologist**

↓

communication ⟶ **Educator**

Remember To Avoid The Professional Idiocy!

When enlisting the help of professionals to find and treat causes of developmental delay, be sure to choose individuals or institutions that respect your opinions and value your observations. You may need to interview several professionals in each category before you find the right expert. Your goal is to create a partnership with each consultant, to which you bring observations and knowledge of your kid and to which the professional brings knowledge of the In/kidding. You must work together to make the wisest use of these mutual contributions for the benefit of your kid. Remember that neither you nor the professionals know the "truth" about everything!

Here follow descriptions of typical contributions made by professionals within the disciplines of Physicians, Psychologists and Educators:

What Your Physician Must Find Out About Developmental Delay

Since any "sick" organ in the body and many life events can sap kids of energy and diminish brain function, a complete history and physical examination is required to rule out disease. Thoroughness is critical to finding the causes of developmental delay!

Here's a list of categories of risk for developmental delays (adapted from First LR & Palfrey JS[1]):

Problems During Pregnancy

- Mother sick during pregnancy
- Drug abuse/medication effects
- Previous abortion

Causes At Birth

- Complicated delivery
- Low birth weight/Prematurity
- Twins/Triplets/more

Disease/Damage To The Baby

- Convulsions/ Brain bleeding
- Meningitis/Blood infection
- Intense (yellow) jaundice
- Low oxygen/Breathing trouble

Inherited Problems

- Others in the family with "delay"
- Blindness/Deafness
- Chromosome/Gene diseases

Problems After Birth

- Convulsions
- Meningitis/Blood infections
- Recurrent ear infections
- Poor feeding/Poor growth
- Lead poisoning/Other pollutants

Social Problems

- Abuse and neglect
- Limited social/financial support
- Teenage parent
- Single parent
- Mentally retarded parent
- Stressful life events
  - Divorce
  - Death of a parent
  - Unemployment of a parent

Identifying the cause of developmental delay is most important because some conditions hide normal skills and others worsen with time and can even lead to death. Developmental-Behavioral Pediatricians and Child Neurologists are trained to identify causes for developmental delay and to manage and coordinate the investigation. If your physician is not experienced evaluating developmental delay, consider consulting with one of these specialists at this stage.

What The Psychologist Must Find Out About Developmental Delay

After a physician has searched for hidden or progressive physical causes for developmental delay, it's necessary to measure *social*-adaptive competence and *communication* skills. These two components of Age Work, together, comprise the essence of "intelligence."

•*social* skills of Age Work include what kids need to relate to and enjoy the presence of others. These abilities encompass self-help skills, like feeding oneself and personal hygiene. They also include making and playing with friends and role-modeling. Psychologists measure these skills with a number of standardized tests of social maturity.

•*communication* skills of Age Work are all the abilities kids need to convey their desires and understand those of others. It is also through these skills that "intelligence" is expressed. Psychologists measure these abilities with standardized tests of intelligence."

Using *social* and *communication* skills together are what we call "intelligence." We don't usually think of intelligence as relying on *physical* abilities, but to some extent, minimal physical abilities are required since complete paralysis makes intelligence non-communicable. Because tests of intelligence are overly reliant on physical abilities before 3 yrs of age, mental retardation cannot be accurately diagnosed prior to that age. Intelligence is an expression of the physical structure and function of the brain and low intelligence, a form of In/kidding, is never a willful disorder.

Besides measuring "intelligence", psychologists measure "achievement." Achievement testing shows the degree to which kids' capabilities (intelligence) have been utilized; that is, it describes how well kids are able to apply their intelligence to solve problems. This is most useful in predicting academic or school performance. As with intelligence testing, achievement testing is more accurate in school-aged kids that in preschoolers. Though kids' achievement levels cannot exceed their intelligence levels, achievement levels lower than intelligence may be due to either innate causes (In/kidding) or willfulness (Out/kidding).

The difference, if any, between capabilities ("IQ") and achievement defines the goal of a school's remedial curriculum. Without this information, parents and teachers can't identify goals or recognize the success or failure of remedial efforts. Both IQ and Achievement testing are critical measures to define the nature and extent of poor school performance. Accuracy in testing is also critical.

Remember that teachers, even Special Education Teachers, unless they have trained as Clinical Child Psychologists, cannot perform accurate IQ and Achievement tests for initial diagnosis. Rather, they can perform screening tests for tracking the progress of interventions after diagnosis. Unfortunately, many schools short of funds will bypass the Clinical Child

Psychologist and perform less expensive screening tests to conform to the letter of the law rather than the more expensive definitive evaluations.

Remember, too, that Clinical Child Psychologists are not the same as School Psychologists. The former professionals are doctoral level experts with training and experience in testing, counseling and therapy. They are able to recognize hidden conditions that degrade performance on IQ and Achievement tests and attest to the reliability of the measurements. School Psychologists' training and experience in counseling and therapy vary widely. Because of their need to fit the student's needs to the school's curriculum, School Psychologists, unless they have been trained and accredited as Clinical Child Psychologists, are best considered Educators. To achieve the best advocacy for your kid's needs, be sure the initial diagnostic testing of IQ and Achievement levels is performed by a Clinical Child Psychologist.

What Educators Do For Kids With Developmental Delay

The most effective means of measuring skill growth in all areas of Age Work, especially for kids with developmental delay, is enrollment in an appropriate (pre)school curriculum where observations of kids' performance can be made over extended periods of time. The professionals best trained to monitor performance, remediate delays and help distinguish developmental delay from progressive disease or mental retardation are Educators.

Educators include not only teachers, but also professionals who assess and exercise each component of the learning process. Here follows a list of Educators whose assistance is of critical importance in each area of Age Work for kids with developmental delay:

physical delays-

- Perceptual Motor Specialists
- Occupational Therapists ⎱ Help kids learn to use their bodies
- Physiotherapists

- Speech & Language Pathologists help kids develop intelligible speech.
- Pupil Personnel Workers ⎱ Assess nutrition and family dynamics
  and
- Social Workers   access community resources.
- Special Education Teachers incorporate interventions into the school curriculum and monitor performance.

social delays-

- School Psychologists track kids' emotional progress and help design Individual Educational Programs (IEP's).

- Pupil Personnel Workers help families cope with disabilities and find community resources.

- Special Education Teachers nurture kids and help them compensate for disabilities.

communication delays-

- Speech & Language Pathologists teach kids alternative methods of communication and enhance language development.

- Learning Disability Teachers help kids acquire and utilize information with techniques that compensate for areas of weakness.

Educators, along with parents, are often the first to observe plateaus of skill development or even the loss of previously attained skills. These observations can truly be life-saving for kids with hidden or poorly managed medical conditions. Here are two examples:

- Kids with PKU, a hereditary metabolic disorder controlled by strict avoidance of a dietary nutrient (phenylalanine), may become irritable and lose previously attained skills if the diet is not being followed at home or at school. Educators, picking up on changes in performance, can alert parents and physicians to the need for better dietary management.

- Kids with Epilepsy, usually well-controlled on anticonvulsants, may "breakthrough" their medications without having visible seizures. Educators may be the only professionals to recognize drops in performance, alerting parents and physicians of the need for a change in medical management.

- Kids with Bipolar Disorder, previously stable under psychiatric care, may trigger an alert from Educators when a sudden deterioration in interpersonal relationships is observed by Educators in the school setting, thus prompting reassessment and adjustment of therapy.

Do Kids Ever Outgrow Developmental Delay?

Yes! Some kids have very exaggerated "normal" variations in development and are "delayed" for brief periods. Others compensate for impairments spontaneously or through medical interventions or educational remediation and catch up fully.

1. First LF, Palfrey JS. The Infant Or Young Child With Developmental Delay (based on standards outlined by Simeonsson and Sharp, Shalowitz and Gorski, and Illingworth. NEJM 1994:478-483.

CHAPTER TWELVE

EPILEPSY & "BEHAVIORAL" SEIZURES

What Is Epilepsy?

Epilepsy is a term describing uncontrolled firing of electrical impulses by brain cells occurring repeatedly, resulting in a temporary disruption of normal brain function and without known cause. Once an epileptic event begins, the *mis*/kidding observed during its occurrence is called a "seizure" and is a form of In/kidding because it is not under a kid's control.

There are different types of seizures:

•**Partial (or "focal") seizures** begin in one discrete place in the brain. When they remain in that place, a kid remains conscious, though not completely functional. Seizures that remains localized to one place in the brain and do not cause unconsciousness are called **"Simple" Partial Seizures**. Simple Partial Seizures, since they allow kids to remain conscious, can be very difficult to recognize, especially if they occur infrequently. Most often, they are *mis*takenly interpreted by parents, teachers, policemen and other observers as willful disobedience.

The tip-off that a Simple Partial Seizure is a form of In/kidding is (as described in Chapter Three):

It qualifies as *Mis*/kidding that affects AGE WORK and-

"*looks*" -	and	"*feels*"-
• *non-selective*		**Confusing**
• *unpredictable*		or
• *of no benefit*		**Anxiety**-provoking

One characteristic of all types of seizures that distinguishes them from Out/kidding (which, as you recall, is willful *mis*/kidding) is their stereotypic nature. This means that seizures, by their very nature, follow the same "script" every time they occur. No matter the circumstances or environment, each seizure event is very much the same as every other seizure event. By contrast, when kids are choosing forms of *mis*/kidding that resemble seizures they cannot reproduce the same, specific movements or actions time after time. Inconsistency between one seizure-like event and another always suggests willful Out/kidding.

When seizures begin in a discrete part of the brain and then spread to the whole brain, consciousness is lost and such seizures are called "generalized" or **"Complex" Partial Seizures**.

•**Generalized or Complex Seizures** begin over the whole brain and cause loss of consciousness from the start. These types of seizures conform to most people's concept of "Epilepsy" and are easily recognized as In/kidding.

Neurologists have names for many other subdivisions of seizures, depending on the part of the brain involved at different stages of seizure progression and the observed effects on kids' functioning.

Most often, seizures include twitching of muscles and are easily recognized. Sometimes though, seizures may exclude muscle twitching and cause internal disruption of kids' normal functions without muscle movements. Such seizures are not easily recognized by the untrained observer. Occasionally, even trained observers may overlook the presence of such "behavioral" seizures, thinking the observed strange or frightening actions are volitional *mis*/kidding. This is the reason it is critical to follow the diagnostic steps of the *Mis*/kidding Process before attempting to solve a *mis*/kidding problem:

- •Determine if the kidding is really *mis*/kidding – Chapter One
- •Determine the severity of the *mis*/kidding – Chapter Two
- •Identify the presence of In/kidding – Chapter Three
  - oThis is where Epilepsy and "behavioral" seizures hide
  - oYou will need professional help to solve this *mis*/kidding

Is Epilepsy Always In/kidding?

Epileptic seizures are always In/kidding because they are not under kids' control. However, epileptic seizures can be triggered by events kids *can* control, such as low blood sugar (as with a diabetic who refuses to take insulin), dehydration (as with not drinking adequate fluids), drug abuse (as with glue sniffing) and extremes of emotion (as when a kid chooses to have a temper tantrum). Many other potential triggers have been identified that kids can control and which can provoke epileptic seizures. In these instances, Out/kidding leads to In/kidding.

As you've learned in Chapter Three, Out/kidding is *mis*/kidding over which kids have control, and its significance is that kids' are making inappropriate choices. As you've also learned, when you're faced with *mis*/kidding that has both In/kidding and Out/kidding components, it's best to identify and treat the In/kidding component first, thus restoring to your kid total control of good/kidding choices. Remember, to identify and treat In/kidding, you will need to get professional help in this order:

Physician ⟶ *Psychologist* ⟶ *Educator*

Once In/kidding is identified and controlled, the Out/kidding component can be dealt with as described in Chapters Four and Five.

What Causes Epilepsy?

Because seizures are caused by the uncontrolled firing of electrical impulses in the brain, any condition or process that triggers such firing can lead to a seizure. Here follows a list of common conditions that can cause seizures:

- Scars in the brain, either from birth or later in life
- Abnormal salt and water balance in the body, as with dehydration
- Inflammation in the brain, as with infections like meningitis
- Areas in the brain with more or less electrical activity, as with tumors
- Chemical effects, as with substance abuse
- High fevers
- Low blood sugar (as with too much insulin)
- Diseases that destroy brain tissue

Having a seizure as a result of one of the above conditions does not mean a kid has epilepsy. For a diagnosis of epilepsy to be made, a kid must have *repeated seizures without known cause*. Such a kid will then be more vulnerable to the effects of any of the above listed conditions and is more likely, as an epileptic, to have a seizure when any such condition is superimposed.

Kids with epilepsy differ from other kids because seizures may be triggered by events to which non-epileptic kids are more resistant. Typical triggers include:

- Hyperventilation, in which kids change the acidity of their blood by breathing too deeply or too rapidly

- Stress, such as anxiety or depression, which can alter brain electrical activity

- Sleep deprivation, which increases brain cell irritability

- Fever, which also increases brain cell irritability

- Flashing lights (including video games!)

- Chemical fumes, as with glue sniffing

How Is Epilepsy Diagnosed?

Not all seizures are "epileptic" and not all forms or epilepsy cause muscle-twitching seizures. The single most commonly used test for identifying epilepsy is a positive ElectroEncephaloGram (EEG or "brainwave" test), observed during a seizure. However, not all epileptic seizures produce easily measured, positive EEG's. When seizures originate in deep areas of the brain, the electrical disturbances may mingle with overlying normal impulses and remain indistinguishable from "normal" brain activity. In these cases, only deep probes, placed during brain surgery, would expose their presence. Sometimes, the mere difficulty of getting a kid to sleep during an EEG recording allows normal waking brain activity to mask an otherwise positive EEG.

You can see how it might be possible for Simple Partial Seizures, occurring deep in the brain and causing *Mid*/kidding or even *KILLER*/kidding, to be ascribed to a psychiatric condition when, in fact, a form of epilepsy might be present. Behavioral manipulations, including behavioral strategies, counseling and psychotherapy would all fail to solve the *mis*/kidding problem because epilepsy, accurately diagnosed or not, is In/kidding and is not under kids' control. Only medical treatment of the seizures would resolve the issue.

Sometimes, tests that do not rely on brain surgery to measure deep-seated origins of seizures are used to rule out the possibility of epilepsy. One such procedure is the Video-Monitored EEG (VME). With this test, *mis*/kidding is documented with a video recording while a simultaneous recording is made of EEG activity. If *mis*/kidding occurs without an abnormality on EEG, the assumption is made that the *mis*/kidding is non-epileptic. The VME suffers from the same limitation as the EEG itself. If the abnormal electrical activity of a deep-seated seizure cannot be "seen" by the EEG, the test will yield a false-negative result.

In order to diagnose some of the conditions which can cause seizures and which were listed earlier in this chapter, other tests, including blood and urine determinations, scans of the head and neck and spinal taps may be performed.

More about "Behavioral" Seizures

Seizures may originate in any part of the brain. Depending on the site of the electrical misfiring in the brain, *mis*/kidding of almost any variety can occur. For example, Simple Partial Seizures (localized, no loss of consciousness) in the temporal lobes of the brain (sides of the brain, at the level of the ears) or frontal lobes (front of the brain) may cause odd sensations or strange acts and may mimic such psychiatric conditions as Obsessive Compulsive Disorder (OCD), Oppositional Defiant Disorder (ODD) and even Schizophrenia. Likewise, Simple Partial Seizures of the limbic system (emotional centers of the brain) may result in rage episodes and other emotional disturbances, easily misdiagnosed as psychiatric conditions.

Seizure-like *mis*/kidding with negative EEG's and negative VME's are often called pseudoseizures or Psychogenic Non-Epileptic Seizures (PNES). When PNES assume the character of rage episodes, they may be diagnosed by Psychiatrists as Intermittent Explosive Disorder. PNES may also resemble the mood cycling of Bipolar Disorder.

How Are Epilepsy, Seizure Disorders & "Behavioral" Seizures Treated?

By definition, "Epilepsy" has no known cause. Seizures caused by known underlying conditions are termed "Seizure Disorders" and, as noted above, seizure-like events unassociated with identifiable EEG abnormalities are termed "PNES." Because EEG's are not 100% reliable, the demarcation between Epilepsy and PNES is somewhat smudged. As a result, the treatment of *mis*/kidding taking the form of seizures is also somewhat indistinct.

Epilepsy and seizure disorders are most commonly treated with medications that increase the threshold for electrical firing of brain cells. Depending on the type of seizures diagnosed, usually on the basis of the abnormal EEG pattern, different medications are known to be most effective. These medications, known as anticonvulsants, when given in high doses, may all cause fatigue as well as other side effects. Often, several anticonvulsants must be used together to adequately control seizures.

For some types of seizures, when anticonvulsants are inadequate for control, severe diet or even brain surgery may be required.

Because the demarcation between epilepsy and PNES is somewhat smudged, several professional helpers may be required to treat the *mis*/kidding of these "Behavioral" Seizures.

What Physicians Do For Behavioral Seizures

As you've learned previously, the qualities of *mis*/kidding that suggest the presence of In/kidding, and specifically epilepsy or a seizure disorder are as follow:

Mis/kidding that suggests **In**/kidding affects AGE WORK and-

"**looks**" -	and	"**feels**"-
• non-selective		**Confusing**
• unpredictable		or
• of no benefit		**Anxiety**-provoking
• **stereotypic**		

By non-selective, we mean kids exhibit the *mis*/kidding randomly. That is, no one person is targeted to the exclusion of all others. By unpredictable, we mean that the *mis*/kidding occurs at random times. The *mis*/kidding doesn't seem to benefit the kids, even from their own perspective. Because of these characteristics, an observer is Confused as to any apparent purpose of the *mis*/kidding and Anxious for the well-being or safety of the kids or others. Finally, the observation most suggestive of epilepsy or a seizure disorder is the stereotypic nature of the *mis*/kidding – its repetitive, unchanging character.

A Pediatrician is the first professional helper to consult if you suspect *mis*/kidding to be In/kidding. When In/kidding takes the form of seizures, this primary care physician will investigate possible causes, including metabolic disorders, substance abuse, dementing illnesses, tumors and other potential underlying diagnoses. EEG's, urine and blood tests, brain scans, lumbar puncture ("spinal tap") and possibly other determinations may be ordered.

Underlying causes of seizure disorders, such as brain tumors and metabolic diseases, often require other, more specialized physicians to become involved, either for more specific diagnoses or for specialized treatments. If no obvious cause for the seizures can be determined, a Child Neurologist may be consulted to distinguish Epilepsy from Psychogenic Non-Epileptic Seizures (PNES). At this point, a Video-Monitored EEG (VME) may be performed in an attempt to observe abnormal brain activity occurring simultaneously with the *mis*/kidding.

When no underlying physical condition or abnormal brain activity can be identified on EEG as a cause for seizures, a diagnosis of PNES is likely to be made. This does not mean a subtle or hidden form of seizure disorder cannot possibly exist. It merely means that reasonable efforts at finding a physical cause for seizure-like episodes have been unsuccessful. In some cases where the observed *mis*/kidding conforms in character to In/kidding, as when the "seizures" are repetitive, stereotypic and resistant to anticonvulsant medications, referral may be made to a Neurosurgeon for more invasive diagnostic tests.

As you will see further on in this chapter, the distinction between a seizure disorder and PNES is not a critical determination for the medical treatment of either condition. Both Neurologists and Psychiatrists share many of the medications used to treat both disorders.

Here follows a list of some anticonvulsants commonly used by Neurologists to treat Epilepsy and Seizure Disorders. You will soon see that Psychiatrists also draw, in part, from this list to treat PNES:

Some Anticonvulsants Commonly Used To Control Epilepsy & Seizure Disorders

- Carbamazepine

- Lamotrigine

- Divalproex

- Oxcarbazepine

- Ethosuccimide

- Topiramate

- Gabapentin

Many other anticonvulsants are also used, depending on the type of seizures being treated, a kid's tolerance for one or another and the "mix" of other medications being prescribed. Though the mechanisms of action of these drugs are beyond the scope of this book, suffice it to say that these medications all decrease the propagation of nerve impulses. As a result, all on the list can be associated with drowsiness and diminished alertness.

What Child Psychiatrists Do For PNES & "Behavioral" Seizures

Child Psychiatrists are usually the professionals of choice for evaluating and treating kids with PNES and Behavioral Seizures. In part, that's because Child Psychiatrists are adept at distinguishing In/kidding from Out/kidding and, in the case of Out/kidding, developing kids' insight and motivation to control destructive choice-making. Also, Child Psychiatrists are familiar with medications and procedures (like ElectroConvulsive Therapy –

[ECT]) that can alter brain function and restore a degree of normalcy to In/kidding.

Among the many conditions Child Psychiatrists treat, most exhibit both an underlying In/kidding component and a superimposed Out/kidding component. One example of such a condition is Intermittent Explosive Disorder (IED). IED is characterized by aggressive, assaultive or destructive episodes occurring out of proportion to a triggering event and not explained by any other known, underlying physical or psychiatric condition[1]. Although by definition IED is not considered a Seizure Disorder, the occurrence of a rage episode may be preceded by many of the same preliminary sensations ("aura") experienced by epileptics before a classic seizure occurs. Clearly, some of the same underlying mechanisms of brain abnormality are common to both conditions. This observation provides a rationale for Child Psychiatrists' use of anticonvulsants in treating IED and Behavioral Seizures.

Although rage episodes in IED are not willful events and therefore cannot be controlled by motivation alone, anger leading to rage is a trigger that an affected kid can learn to control. This dual nature of the *mis*/kidding of IED requires the Psychiatrist not only to develop a kid's coping mechanisms through counseling and therapy to avoid triggering rage through anger, but also reducing brain vulnerability to rage, usually with medication.

Beside anger as a trigger for "Behavioral" Seizures, anxiety and depression are frequent companions to PNES and "Behavioral" Seizures. To reduce the In/kidding component of these forms of *mis*/kidding, Psychiatrists may prescribe antianxiety, antidepressant or antipsychotic medications, either singly or in combination.

Here follow three groups of medications commonly used by Psychiatrists to control "Behavioral" Seizures in kids. There are other drugs, less commonly used or newly developed, that are not listed below. Note that some of the anticonvulsants already introduced to you were mentioned in the treatment of Epilepsy and Seizure Disorders by Neurologists earlier in this Chapter.

Medications Commonly Used By Psychiatrists For "Behavioral"

Anticonvulsants	Antidepressants	Antipsychotics
• Carbamazepine	• Buproprion	• Lithium
• Divalproex	• Mirtazapine	• Haldol
• Gabapentin	• Desvenlafaxine	• Risperdone
• Lamotrigine	• Citalopram	• Aripiprazole
• Oxcarbazepine	• Fluoxetine	• Quetiapine
• Topiramate	• Sertraline	• Ziprasidone

Seizures

In addition to anticonvulsants, antidepressants and antipsychotic medications, Psychiatrists may prescribe medications for anxiety, insomnia and drug dependency, all of which conditions can also trigger "Behavioral" Seizures.

Psychiatrists are often part of a team of professionals who diagnose, treat and monitor "Behavioral" Seizures. They often depend on Psychologists to acquire critical measures of kids' performance, implement strategies and provide ongoing counseling and therapy.

What Psychologists Do For Epilepsy and "Behavioral" Seizures

Psychologists, though they are not medical doctors and cannot prescribe medications, are best positioned to track the effects of Epilepsy and other forms of seizures on the intellectual capabilities and performance of kids. Both Seizure Disorders themselves and the effects of the medications used to treat them impact on the Consequence Areas of Age Work and the relationships kids have to Others and Authority. In other words, Psychologists can measure the success or failure of treatment strategies by tracking changes in *mis*/kidding.

Some of the basic tools Psychologists use to measure kids' progress include IQ tests, Achievement tests and measures of Social Maturity. IQ tests measure what kids *can* do. Achievement tests measure what kids *are doing*. Tests of Social Maturity measure how much kids know about what they *should be doing*. These are the critical components of "psychometrics" or "mind measures."

These tests are usually fun for kids to take because they are presented in a play format, especially for younger kids and because there are no "grades" given to kids. Rather, results are presented as "age equivalents" (also called mental age), "percentiles" (comparisons to the normal level) or "grade equivalents" (hypothetical "guesstimate" of the school grade a kid can handle in that skill area). Psychiatrists, parents, teachers and other caretakers can easily understand and utilize these *interchangeable* results in judging the effectiveness of treatment. Scores can be compared from one time to another so that loss of skills can be recognized, if they are occurring and gains in performance documented when treatment is effective.

Psychometrics performed by Psychologists are not the same as academic testing by teachers. Psychologists perform extensive (and time-consuming) tests and they are trained to account for kids "having a bad day", such as when kids haven't taken their medications or when kids are experiencing headache or other confounding circumstances. Tests performed by teachers are Achievement Tests and as noted above, measure only what kids are doing, while tests by Psychologists can measure both what kids are doing and what kids are capable of doing. Sometimes schools use Achievement Tests by teachers to plan special programs or services because such tests take less time and are less expensive to perform than formal psychometrics. Because such tests take into account only what kids are doing for whatever reason, rather than what they could do if they were working at their ability level, such tests can "fulfill their own prophesies." Individualized Educational Plans (IEP's) based on such tests may accept low levels of performance as "normal" for a kid whose abilities are much higher. The result may be a kid who fails to advance academically or who becomes either bored or confused by the curriculum only to engage in more intense *mis*/kidding.

Besides testing kids, Psychologists can provide the necessary therapy and counseling services needed to overcome Out/kidding. They can advise Educators of kids' specific capabilities and needs as a basis for appropriate IEP's.

What Educators Do For Epilepsy and "Behavioral" Seizures

Educators, equip kids with many of the skills they need to flourish in "real life." When kids have special needs, Educators can construct Individualized Educational Programs (IEP's) to overcome otherwise disabling physical and psychiatric disorders like Epilepsy and "Behavioral" Seizures. Because Educators observe kids for half their waking hours much of the week, they are well positioned to make critical observations of kids' responses to treatment strategies and measure their progress. Here are some of the Educators that can help your kid. Their designations vary from state to state:

- Principals (and Vice Principals) oversee the delivery of school services, but they also have authority to intercede when bullying is an issue.

- Teachers act as the "eyes and ears" for those professionals whose treatments are in play, but who cannot be "on-site."

- Special Education Teachers can build on kids' strengths, helping them compensate for areas of weakness.

- School Counselors can help kids acquire coping skills and develop social proficiency.

- Physical and Occupational Therapists (sometimes called Perceptual Motor Specialists) also assist kids acquire social skills, but can strengthen physical competency as well.

- Educational Specialists (math, speech and language, reading) assist kids in academic areas of need, closing gaps between capabilities and achievement levels.

- Audiologists monitor kids' hearing ability and assess aids to hearing.

- Social Workers (sometimes called Pupil Personnel Workers) can assist kids and their families to acquire additional resources, both financial and professional, to achieve treatment goals.

- School Nurses can administer medications during school hours, monitor their effects and transmit observations to the prescribing physicians.

- School Psychologists (sometimes called Educational Psychologists, Psychometrists) can provide "on-site" counseling for such *mis*/kidding as anger flare-ups and the management of bullying. They can also determine kids' capabilities and compare their levels of achievement with those capabilities. Discrepancies between capabilities and achievement levels define the educational goals of an IEP.

Medications used to control Epilepsy, PNES and "Behavioral" Seizures may blunt alertness or cause other side effects which impact on learning and social relationships. Often, such side effects are weighed by prescribing physicians against the anticipated benefits of the medications. Perhaps the most important contribution Educators make to the management of Epilepsy, Seizure Disorders and PNES acting as the "eyes and ears" of prescribing physicians, providing a basis for dose adjustments or alternative treatments.

References:

1.Impulse-Control Disorders: Diagnostic Criteria from DSM-IV-TR, Am. Psych. Assoc. 2000

Appendix I

Critical Markers for Age Work

You have learned that the first three steps to change *mis*/kidding to good/kidding are:

1.   Identifying *mis/*kidding

2.   Limiting the *mis/*kidding to *Mid/*kidding   "Diagnostic" Phase

3.   Eliminating any *In/*kidding

Because In/kidding presents physical barriers to choice-making, its presence will limit a kid's compliance with A/L Commands. Indeed, some forms of In/kidding, like Autistic Spectrum Disorders, AD(H)D, Bipolar Disorder, Cerebral Palsy, Developmental and Intellectual Disabilities and Epilepsy, force us to accept or adjust to degrees of *mis*/kidding. Thus, Step 3, eliminating In/kidding, must be achieved to insure success with the management phase of the *Mis*/kidding Process.

To eliminate In/kidding, and with it any barriers to a kid's free choice-making, we must be sure the kid can meet age-related expectations within the *physical, social* and *communication* ability areas of AGE WORK. It is not necessary to consult a specialist before making this determination. Some simple "markers" in each skill area are sufficient for you to decide if In/kidding is likely. Only if and when a kid fails to meet one or more markers of delayed AGE WORK, suggesting the presence of In/kidding over which the kid has no control, would professional assistance be required. Such assistance, you may recall, would follow this path:

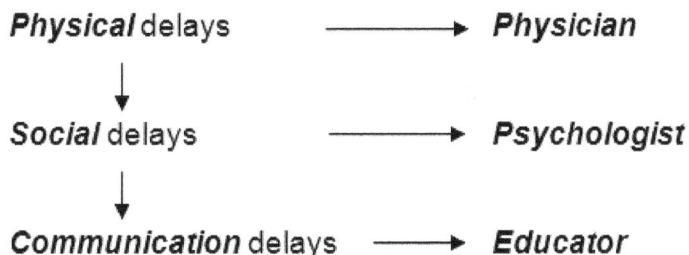

Physical delays   ⟶   **Physician**

↓

Social delays   ⟶   **Psychologist**

↓

Communication delays   ⟶   **Educator**

The assistance you seek from an expert in each of these disciplines consists of finding out possible causes for the delay, eliminating any potentially health-threatening or progressive conditions causing the delay and measuring your kid's "baseline" performance for future comparison. Measuring baselines is critical for identifying your kid's response to medical, psychological or educational interventions. Without such initial measures, you will not be able to judge the success or failure of the experts' proposed treatments or identify conditions that worsen your kid's performance.

Tell Me Again – What Services Must I Get From The Professional?

When you seek professional assistance to evaluate delays in Age Work, you must specifically request answers to these three sets of questions:

- What are the possible causes of the delay and how will they be identified or eliminated?

- Will any of the possible causes of the delay result in a "leveling off" or even a loss of progress and if that happens, how will it be recognized?

- At what level is your kid currently functioning and how far from "normal" is that level at this time? Also, what tests will be given to track progress and how often will they be administered.

Any professional who cannot or will not answer these questions in a direct and easily understood fashion is the wrong expert for your kid.

Here follows a compilation of suggested "markers" for various age ranges in each of the skill areas of AGE WORK. It represents indices of kids' competence which I have observed and found useful over many years of Behavioral Pediatric practice. These markers are not meant to be used as the sole measure of intelligence or developmental age. Rather, they are presented for the purpose of recognizing delays in Age Work that point to In/kidding and which might block your management of *mis*/kidding. This is a reference you can use to quickly check for delays in AGE WORK that make you

Is *observed* to be-	or	Makes you *feel-*
• Unpredictable or random		Anxious
		or
• Of no benefit to the kid		Confused
• Threatening		

suspicious of In/kidding. You will look here whenever *Mid*/kidding:

To use this Appendix, find your kid's age range and see if the "markers" are met for *physical, social* and *communication* abilities for that age range. If so, In/kidding is unlikely and your kid is free to choose good/kidding; thus you may continue on to the management steps of the *Mis*/kidding Process. If not, your kid may need evaluation, diagnosis and possible treatment for In/kidding. And sometimes you may discover you'll have to limit your expectations accordingly.

See chart on the next page.

Markers of *Age Work* For Various Age Ranges [1,2]

Note: *Markers for Age Work are coded to indicate which professionals to consult first if delays are suspected-*

"ꝑ" *Physician*   "♥" *Psychologist*   "⌂" *Educator*

	Physical	Social	Communication
Newborn Baby	ꝑ Moves all extremities ꝑ Sucks to feed ꝑ Passes urine and stool	ꝑ Able to calm when held and rocked	ꝑ Able to cry loudly
By 3 months	ꝑ Lifts head up when lying on belly ꝑ Able to unclench fists ꝑ Reacts to visual threat	ꝑ Anticipates feeding ꝑ Recognizes parent ꝑ Able to smile	ꝑ Coos "musically"
By 5 months	ꝑ Able to hold rattle ꝑ Can roll over to back	ꝑ Smiles socially	ꝑ Able to babble
By 6 months	ꝑ Sits alone briefly ꝑ Can suck toes ꝑ Transfers objects from one hand to other ꝑ Reaches for objects	ꝑ Recognizes someone is a stranger ꝑ Feeds self ꝑ Searches for toy	ꝑ Turns to voice ꝑ Single syllables
By 8 months	ꝑ Sits without support	ꝑ Laughs in playful situations	ꝑ Able to say "da", "ba"
By 9 – 10 months	ꝑ Able to crawl ꝑ Pulls to standing ꝑ Walks holding on	ꝑ Explores environment ꝑ Plays pat-a-cake ꝑ Indicates wants	ꝑ Understands "No!" ꝑ Says "Mama, Dada" (Non-specific)
By 12 months	ꝑ Stands alone briefly ꝑ Walks alone briefly ꝑ Picks up small objects	♥ Imitates activities ♥ Cooperates with dressing	ꝑ Says "Mama, Dada" (Specific) ꝑ Follows one step commands w/ gesture
By 15 months	ꝑ Creeps up stairs ꝑ Scribbles ꝑ Stacks 2 blocks	ꝑ Drinks from a cup ♥ "Helps" with housework	♥ At least 4 words
By 18 months	ꝑ Runs ꝑ Throws while standing ꝑ Turns pages in a book	♥ Plays alongside other kids ♥ Uses spoon and fork	♥ Knows 5 body parts ♥ Knows at least 6 words

Markers of *Age Work* For Various Age Ranges[1,2] (Continued)

Note: Markers for Age Work are coded to indicate which professionals to consult first if delays are suspected-

"ᵽ" *Physician*   "♥" *Psychologist*   "⚖" *Educator*

	Physical	Social	Communication
By 2 years age	ᵽ Walks up & down stairs without help ᵽ Can partially undress ᵽ Imitates pencil strokes	♥ Brushes teeth with help ♥ Imitates washing and drying hands ᵽ Anticipates toileting needs	♥ Uses 2 word phrases ♥ Uses pronouns (I, you, me) *inappropriately* ♥ Follows 2 step commands
By 3 years age	ᵽ Alternates feet when climbing stairs ᵽ Can peddle a tricycle ♥ Copies a circle	♥ Knows name and gender ♥ Shares toys ♥ Washes hands	♥ 3 word phrases ♥ Uses pronouns *appropriately* ♥ Uses plurals
By 4 years age	ᵽ Hops, skips, alternates feet going *down* stairs ᵽ Buttons clothes ♥ Copies a square	♥ Plays *cooperatively* with other kids ♥ Dresses without help	ᵽ+♥ Knows colors ♥ Asks questions ⚖ Speech understandable to *everyone*
By 5 years age	ᵽ Able to balance briefly on 1 foot ᵽ Adequate stamina for preschool or K ♥ Able to draw a stick figure of a person	♥ Plays competitively ♥ Abides by rules ♥ Helps with household chores	⚖ Prints 1st name ⚖ Asks meaning of words ♥ Understands opposites
From 6–12 years	ᵽ Passes yearly physical exam by Pediatrician ᵽ Adequate stamina for daily activities	♥ Able to make friends ♥ Enjoys meeting parents' expectations ♥ Maintains personal hygiene	⚖ Achieves within 1 year of grade level in school (for age)
From 13–18 years	ᵽ Passes yearly physical exam by Pediatrician ᵽ Adequate stamina for daily activities	♥ Able to make friends of either sex ♥ Maintains personal hygiene ♥ Controls emotions without threat to Age Work, Others or Authority	⚖ Achieves within 1 grade level in school (for age) *AND/OR* ⚖ Able to retain a job, if of legal age, attending to schedules & work-related duties

1. Age ranges 1 month through 5 years adapted from Table 8-4 <u>The Harriet Lane Handbook</u>, 16th Edition – Mosby.
2. Age ranges 1 month through 6 years adapted from <u>Denver Developmental Assessment (Denver II)</u> – Univ Colorado Medical School 1990.

*Age ranges 1 month through 5 years adapted from Table 8-4 The Harriet Lane Handbook, 16th Edition – Mosby.

**Age ranges 1 month through 6 years adapted from Denver Developmental Assessment (Denver II) – University of Colorado Medical School, 1990.

CAUTION: For kids up to two years of age who were prematurely born, chronological or "real" age must be corrected before it can be used to plot developmental milestones. This is done by subtracting the number of months of prematurity from "real" age. For example:

An eighteen month old kid was born after thirty weeks of pregnancy.

"Normal" pregnancy = 40 wks

This kid's pregnancy = 30 wks

Number of weeks premature =10 wks

(Divide by 4 to convert to months = 2.5 months

This toddler's chronological ("real") age = 18 mos

Number of months prematurity = -2.5 mos

"Corrected" chronological age = 15.5 mos

This is the age used to find expected milestones or "markers" in the table above. After two years of age, this correction is not necessary.

What to Do If You Find Delays in Age Work & Your Physician Says, "The Kid Will Grow Out Of It"?

If you've determined your kid is *KILLER*/kidding, STOP IT IMMEDIATELY, if you can. If you need a professional's assistance and yours is unwilling to help, *find another* professional to assist you. Don't engage in the Professional Idiocy – remember that no one, including professionals, knows the TRUTH about everything!

If delay is at the *mini*/kidding level, follow your professional's advice and wait to see if your kid outgrows it. Once delays in Age Work are confined to the *Mid*/kidding level and are being monitored by the corresponding professionals, you need to track your kid's progress with the experts.

Though most professionals are committed to providing the best possible care, no professional can be as diligent as a loving parent. Limitations imposed by medical insurance, client "overload" and school budgets can delay or even obstruct the process of monitoring your kid's progress and the provision of critical services by physicians, psychologists or educators. You must track your kid's developmental delays so that you can judge how well or how poorly the interventions are working, whether your kid is gaining or losing ground and whether other approaches are needed.

How to Track Kids' Development in Any Skill Area of Age Work

From each professional who has measured "baseline" skills for your kid and has confirmed delays, ask for a short list of "marker" skills your kid has demonstrated at that age. You should be able to find most of them in the table above. If the testing is accurate, you will quickly recognize the delays you have already observed (and which prompted you to get help initially). If you have seen your kid perform at a higher level than the tests indicate, don't engage in the Professional Idiocy! Inform the professional of the discrepancy and arrange retesting. If you lack confidence in that professional, insist on retesting by another expert. Second opinions bolster confidence in test results and provide a more solid basis for time-consuming or costly interventions.

Once you have a short list of observed skills from the testing (or from your own observations), you can mark those skills on a graph as shown below to see how far from "normal" your kid is performing now. Each time new testing is done, ask for a few more "markers" of accomplishment. Plotting these over time will show whether your kid is "closing the gap", maintaining a plateau or losing ground. Though this sounds complicated, it's actually very easy to do. Here's how:

How to Construct "Normal" Charts to Monitor Your Kid's Progress

Begin by drawing a chart of "normal" skill growth. You'll use this to follow your kid's progress in any (or all) skill areas of Age Work over time. Be sure the ages you plot extend from the lowest level of performance your kid has demonstrated in testing to several years beyond your kid's "real" age. Imagine, for example, your kid is 2 yrs old. Your graph might extend from a newborn's age (0 yrs) to 4 years of age. You'd be able to use this chart till your kid is four years old. I'll show you how to enter test results or your own observations a little further on.

To construct the chart, plot "Apparent" or "Performance" Age on the left and Real" or Chronological" Age on the bottom for the chosen age range:

Here's how the graph looks for skills from 0 years through 4 years of age:

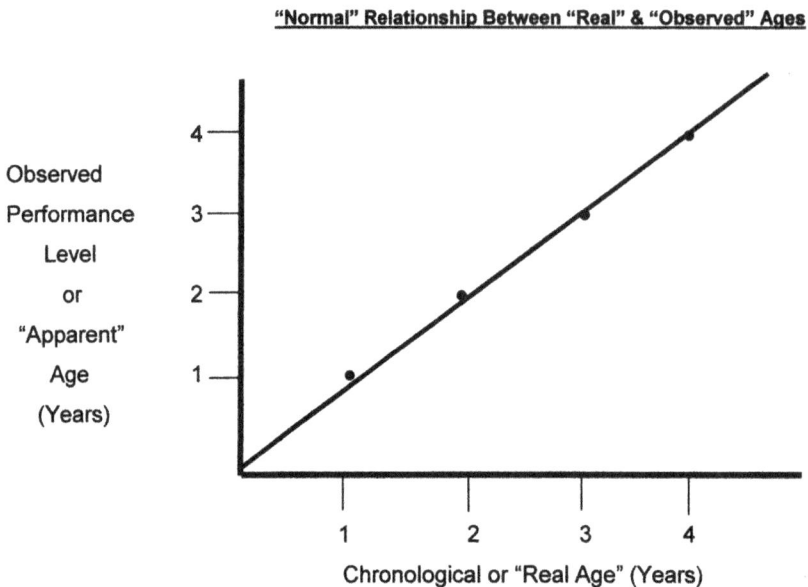

"Normal" Relationship Between "Real" & "Observed" Ages

Observed Performance Level or "Apparent" Age (Years)

Chronological or "Real Age" (Years)

All this chart "says" is that a "normal" kid's "observed" age is at about the same level as the kid's "real" age – neither much above, nor much below that level. That is, one year old kids perform skills that are typically seen at the one year level; two year old kids perform at about the two year level, and so on. This should be no surprise since professionals "standardize" their tests to achieve this relationship.

You'll use this chart to plot your kid's "observed" performance against this "normal" performance in each skill area of Age Work over time. You'll need three copies of this chart – one for each of the three skill areas of Age Work – *physical, social* and *communication*.

Here's how to use the charts:

Using Your Charts To Track Your Kid's Physical Progress

Label each of your charts for the skill area you want to track. For this example, let's choose to track *physical* development for a 4 year old who was recognized as "delayed" at 10 months of age and who has been enrolled in an Infant and Toddler program since 10 months of age.

Here are 4 skills that were first observed at 10 months, 18 months, 3 years and again at 4 years of age:

- Began rolling over from stomach to back at 10 months of age
- Began crawling at 18 months

- Began walking up and down stairs at 3 years of age
- Is now (at 4 years of age) peddling a tricycle

Looking up these skills in our "Markers of Age Work" chart (above), we see they "normally" occur at 5 months, 10 months, 2 yrs and 3 yrs, respectively.

Plotting them on our physical chart, they would look like this:

Four *Physical* Skills Observed (or tested) At 10, 18, 36 and 48 Months

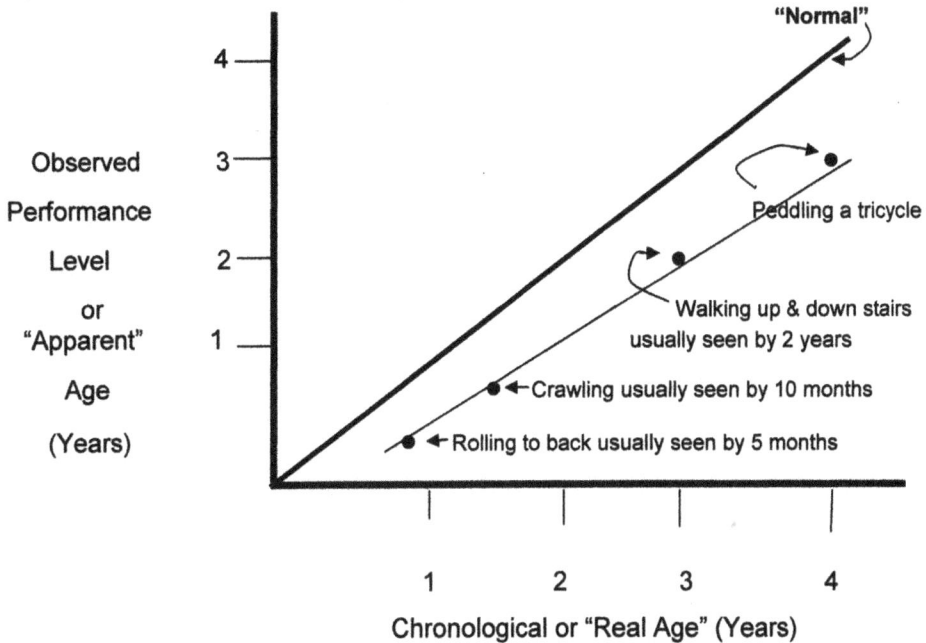

In this example, a kid exhibited developmental delay at 10 months of age. He first started to roll to his back at that age, a physical skill normally seen by 5 months of age. He was then enrolled in a preschool program to monitor and enhance his progress. By 18 months of age, he began to crawl, a skill normally seen by 10 months of age. By 3 years of age, he began walking up and down stairs, a skill normally seen at 2 years of age. Now that he is 4 years old, he is beginning to peddle a tricycle, a skill normally developed by 3 years of age.

When these "markers" are plotted out on our "normal" chart for physical development, we see that this kid is not catching up. Indeed, he may be falling further behind. This type of chart is often seen in kids with Mental Retardation.

If a diagnosis of mental retardation is under consideration for this 4 year old, plotting this type of chart will help parents (and professionals as well) to monitor rates of progress for this kid. But if the parents of this kid were advised by the school that their "developmentally delayed" kid was "doing well" in the program, they would have good reason to question either the adequacy of the program or the accuracy of the professional(s) diagnosis.

Using Your Charts To Track Your Kid's Social Progress

In this example, we'll track the *social* development of a 7 year old kid who was recognized to have delays in that skill area at 2 years of age. Here are 4 social skills that were first observed at 2 years, 3 years, 5 years and now (at 7 years of age):

- First began to laugh at 2 years of age
- Began to cooperate with dressing at 3 years of age
- Began playing alongside other kids at 5 years of age
- Has now (at 7 years of age) begun to respond to his name

Looking up these skills in our "Markers of Age Work" chart (above), we see they "normally" occur at 8 months, 12 months, 18 months and 3 years of age, respectively.

Plotting them on our social chart would look like this:

See chart on the next page.

Four _Social_ Skills Observed (or tested) At 2, 3, 5, and 7 Years of Age

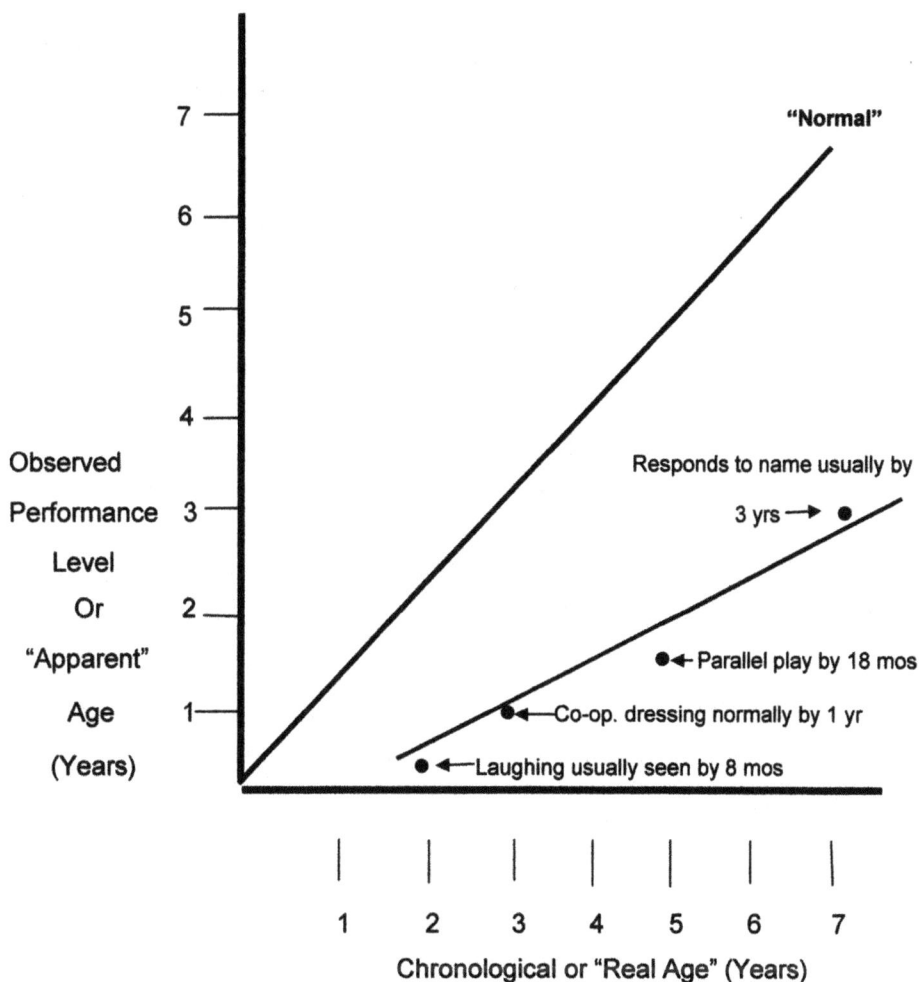

Observed

Performance

Level

Or

"Apparent"

Age

(Years)

"Normal"

Responds to name usually by

3 yrs → ●

●←— Parallel play by 18 mos

●←——Co-op. dressing normally by 1 yr

● ←——Laughing usually seen by 8 mos

1   2   3   4   5   6   7

Chronological or "Real Age" (Years)

On the chart above we see the pattern of delayed _social_ milestones often encountered with kids who are either Mentally Retarded or who suffer from Autism. Kids with Autism and other conditions within the category of Autistic Spectrum Disorders often benefit greatly from educational interventions and such benefit would show up on a chart like this with either a consistent and stable gap or a narrowing gap.

If a diagnosis of Mental Retardation were under consideration for this 7 year old, plotting this type of chart would help to monitor rates of progress for this kid. But seeing an increasingly wide gap between "normal" and a kid's measured or observed pattern of progress, a parent whose kid had been diagnosed with Developmental Delay or an Autistic Spectrum Disorder would have to question either the adequacy of the program or the accuracy of the diagnosis.

Using Your Charts To Track Your Kid's Communication Progress

Now, let's see how we can track a kid's *communication* skills. Since this group of abilities within Age Work includes academic (school) performance, this type of chart will likely be used more often and for a wider range of ages than those for *physical* or *social* skills.

Communication skill charts can (and should) be used to enlighten teachers when report cards claim "satisfactory" progress and parents and/or other professionals fail to see such progress. Especially sensitive to monitoring with these charts are Special Education interventions for Learning Disabilities, since, by definition, such disabilities are remediable with proper classroom assistance. In other words, if it's the wrong class, the wrong teacher or the wrong diagnosis, the chart will graphically demonstrate no "catch-up" or even wider "gaps" over time.

Here are the results of 3 sets of tests administered to a (now) 13 yr old kid diagnosed at 8 years of age with "dyslexia." He is about to be "mainstreamed" to a *Mid*dle School from a Special Education program:

- At 8 yrs of age (3rd grade) he was "reading" at a pre-kindergarten level

- At 10 yrs of age (5th grade) he was reading at a 3rd grade (8 yr) level

- Now, at 13 years of age, he's reading at the 8th grade level

Here's how his communication chart looks: *(see next page)*

Three _Communication_ Skills Tested At 8, 10, and 13 Years of Age

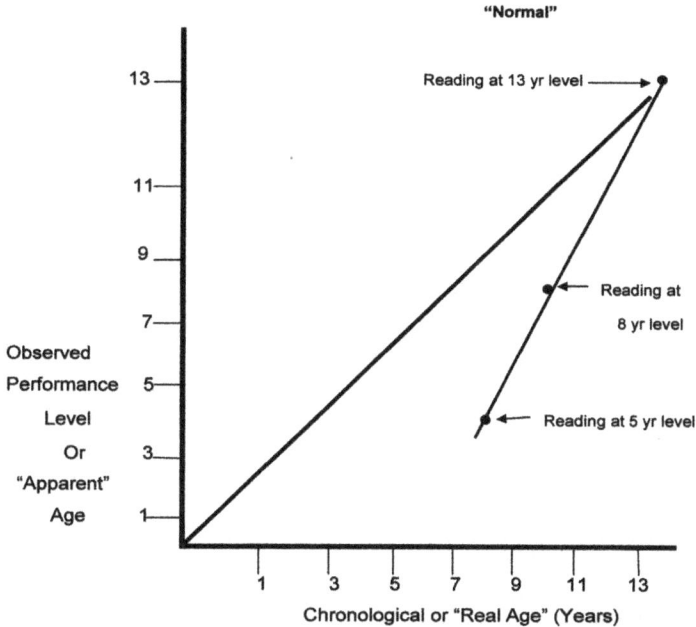

This chart shows a successful remediation of "dyslexia" over a period of five years. The accuracy of the diagnosis and the appropriateness of the school program are not in doubt.

These examples should reassure you that following your kid's progress is an easy task. The charts provide a visual "track" of progress in any or all three areas of Age Work. Specific patterns of performance among the three skill areas are characteristic of certain forms of In/kidding. Indeed, professionals often use charts much like these to diagnose In/kidding.

The most common forms of In/kidding and those most likely to impair kids' choice-making (and so your management of _mis_/kidding) are discussed in detail in Part II of this book.

Appendix II

More Techniques For Kid Control

In the first three chapters of this book you learned to:

- •Recognize *mis*/kidding

- •Isolate *Mid*/kidding by stopping *KILLER*/kidding and to ignore *mini*/kidding, and

- •Get professional help for In/kidding

In Chapters Four and Five you learned how to manage Out/kidding, the inappropriate acts in which kids choose to engage. In Chapter Four you became acquainted with the "wiring" of appropriate good/kidding commands in the Deterrence, Deflection, Diversion or Drawing modes and in Chapter Five you saw how to "energize" those commands with powerful A/L Consequences.

Here it will be helpful to learn some additional "tricks of the trade" to control Out/kidding and promote good/kidding. We'll begin with some Star Chart techniques.

The Positive Reinforcement Star Chart Technique

The Positive Reinforcement Star Chart technique begins with no stars. Kids get stars as successes are achieved. As such, it "wires" good/kidding commands in the Drawing mode, aiming to motivate kids who are passively *mis*/kidding and inducing them to move toward a good/kidding goal. In other words, this is a good technique to use when kids are failing to do what they're supposed to do. You may recall that the Drawing mode "draws" kids toward a reward and presents no risk of evoking anger.

Younger kids, with mental ages between three and ten to twelve years, can't usually visualize or recall goals that are merely spoken or which are achieved over several days or weeks. To make the process of earning rewards for good/kidding more concrete and easily understood, a visual means of tracking their progress with stars allows them to remain motivated and see their "reward" getting closer with each success.

Star (or any simple token) charts "keep score" of kids' progress. Drawings or photos of the rewards kids are working toward can be pasted onto the last box of the charts so that kids "see" what reward lies in store for their success.

Kids with mental ages between three and five years usually do best with only one required act per half day (morning vs. afternoon) for each star. For example, a star in the morning and one in the afternoon for not wetting pants. More complexity is usually not well understood. Remember that a "star" is really only a "token" of success, but it does represent what might be called a "minisuccess" and achieving a star should be accompanied by lots of praise to make it "feel" like a minisuccess.

Young kids do even better remembering their goal when a reward can be seen, touched and played with before starting a star chart. A trip to the toy store, where a kid can play with the proposed reward briefly, then returning it to the shelf and coming home (with the kid undoubtedly screaming!) will "fix" the reward in a kid's mind, giving more meaning to the stars that lead to the reward. A photo taken in the store with a cell phone and then pasted to the star chart identifies the actual reward "waiting for you to get your stars."

Young kids do best with daily rewards for up to two stars per day. For older kids, star charts can have several rows for each of several days. Kids with older mental ages than five years may not need a trip to the store and will usually do well talking about the goal, then writing it into the last box on the chart. For example, at age ten, three stars might be required each day for several days to acquire the reward. One star might be given for "being kind to your brother", another for "cleaning your room" and a third for "doing your homework."

The key to success with a star chart is not the stars; it's the choice of the reward that seduces the kid to perform a difficult task. As you've learned in Chapter Four, "things", though potentially effective, are not as powerful rewards as affection or, when doled out by a loved one, Superaffection. For example, two stars might be required by the end of the day to eat with the family instead of eating alone in one's room.

Positive Reinforcement Star Charts require kids to experience rewards before they become "hooked" on their success. This process of "drawing" kids to rewards avoids triggering anger, but it takes a bit longer than somewhat more punitive strategies. Let's look next at the Negative Reinforcement Star Chart.

The Negative Reinforcement Star Chart

Negative Reinforcement Star Charts begin with kids having possession of an adequate number of stars to complete a successful day, or sometimes, extra stars. Each *mis*/kidding episode results in the loss of a star. At the end of specified periods, as for example, AM, then PM, remaining stars are affixed to the chart and new stars are given for the next sequence. Kids, when they are "short" of a required number of stars, must work "extra" (perform more good/kidding) to earn more stars and get their reward. Usually, a kid is given stars to carry in a pocket. If the targeted *mis*/kidding is observed, a warning may be given, after which, if the *mis*/kidding persists, a star is taken away.

The Negative Reinforcement Star Chart presents kids with both the opportunity to earn rewards by retaining their stars and the risk of losing their stars and thus their rewards. This dual presentation of a potential reward or punishment "wires" good/kidding commands in the Deflection mode. The potential punishment of losing a star "deflects" the kid's *mis*directed energy away from the anticipated *mis*/kidding goal and toward the desired good/kidding reward.

You may recall that presenting Word Language Commands in the "Deflection" mode is the most efficient way to control active *mis*/kidding; that is, situations in which kids are actively doing things they're not supposed to do. Though "wiring" in the "Deflection" mode preserves much of the energy kids devote to *mis*/kidding, the punishment component does evoke some anger which can ricochet back to the caregiver.

An example of the usefulness of a Negative Reinforcement Star Chart is with the *mis*/kidding of bullying within the house. A four year old who bullies his younger sister might be told he will need a morning star and an afternoon star to eat with the family. A chart is posted in his room with the designated open boxes. Stars are given for the kid to carry in his pocket. He is advised he needs to keep his stars for the chart "so you can eat with us." If he is seen bullying his sister, he is given a warning, but if this *mis*/kidding persists, a star is taken from him. At the end of the agreed upon period, stars are affixed to the chart. Open boxes mean eating alone. Such Superaffection denied is an extremely powerful consequence for the *mis*/kidding of bullying.

With this technique, you might begin by estimating how many times each morning and how many times each afternoon the kid engages in the target *mis*/kidding. In the example above, if the kid averages three bullying episodes per half day, three stars might be given in the morning and three in the afternoon. By reducing the *mis*/kidding to two episodes in the morning and two in the evening, the kid would retain one star for each half day, representing a degree of success for that day and earning the reward. The next day, two stars might be given to start each half day, requiring even better control of the *mis*/kidding. Depending on the type of *mis*/kidding being targeted, the rate at which you reduce the number of beginning stars each day might vary, but the principle is the same; a gradual reduction of the *mis*/kidding over time by risking loss of stars while offering rewards for success. The younger the kid, the more important it is to offer a reward for each successful day, since most young kids can't conceptualize the "big picture."

Negative Reinforcement Star Charts risk creating anger because taking away a star is really a direct punishment. Generating anger can work against you, especially if a kid already has anger issues. But when anger has not been a major issue for a kid, Negative Reinforcement Star Charts can be a most effective means of demonstrating your displeasure with specific forms of *mis*/kidding. And when other kids are observing, the technique provides concrete examples to them of "loss" that occurs as a result of *mis*/kidding.

Now, let's examine how you can magnify the power of Star Chart techniques in controlling *mis*/kidding by incorporating sibling rivalry, the normal competition between brothers and sisters for parental Superaffection, to *your* benefit.

Competitive Sibling-Enhanced Star Charts

Sibling rivalry can be used to powerfully energize good/kidding efforts, using either Positive or Negative Reinforcement Star Charts. The technique can be imposed on one of two or more siblings who is engaging in *mis*/kidding, using the other siblings who are good/kidding as the standards to be met. Or, if all the siblings are engaged in *mis*/kidding, a designated number of stars may be required for any of the kids to capture a reward. In the examples to follow, Star Charts provide a means of measuring and acknowledging good/kidding. The competing siblings are motivated by sibling rivalry to overwhelm their *mis*/kidding goals with good/kidding goals.

This technique is so powerful and the withdrawal of Superaffection so painful for some parents to watch, that those who forget the distinction between love and affection are often completely immobilized and unable to effectively utilize the technique. For such parents it is worthwhile to recall the discussion of love and affection presented in Chapter Three. Specifically, that the heritage of love is given to kids no matter if they are *mis*/kidding or good/kidding, but the gift of affection (Superaffection, in the case of a love relationship) is doled out as a reward for good/kidding and, to maintain an honest relationship, withheld when it is undeserved by acts of *mis*/kidding. Honesty, you will recall, along with Nurturance and the imposition of

Responsibility comprise the HoNoR Role for parents, which is critical for kids to grow into successful adults.

To fulfill the HoNoR Role while using Competitive Sibling-Enhanced Star Charts, "the stars must fall where they may", giving the siblings an Honest appraisal of their success in good/kidding, Nurturance, in the form of affection (or Superaffection) as a reward for their achievement and the opportunity to accept Responsibility for the consequences they have earned.

As an example of a Competitive Sibling-Enhanced Star Chart, consider two sisters, aged four and six years. The six year old is fully toilet trained and the four year old intentionally urinates in her clothes, though you know she can tell when she needs to urinate. Indeed, she tells you when she needs to go, then says, "No!" and wets herself when you ask her to go to the bathroom.

You set up a Competitive Sibling-Enhanced Star Chart in the Negative Reinforcement mode. Both sisters are given a star to carry. They are brought to a toy store where each girl chooses a toy as a reward for success, then replaces it on the shelf. At home, a chart is posted with one box for each girl that day. They are advised that "anyone who pees in their clothes will lose her star." At day's end, "Everyone with a star goes back to store and gets their toy." If younger sister wets her clothes, her star is taken and, at day's end, both girls go to the store, but only the older sister gets a toy." It's likely younger sister will come home crying. But, you explain, "We'll do the same thing tomorrow." This powerful technique will usually solve the *mis*/kidding problem within a day or two.

There are variations on this theme. For example, no siblings are required, as shown next.

Competitive Adult-Enhanced Star Charts

Dads and Moms can participate in what could be called Competitive Adult-Enhanced Star Charts. Indeed, the whole family can participate with kids of various ages for different age-related rewards. With these Star Charts it is critical to choose seductive rewards to properly motivate each participant. Star Charts can span days, weeks, even months once all participants are engaged in the process.

As an example, using the vignette presented above, except substituting Mom or Dad for the older sibling, the four year old "wetter" can compete with one or more parents for the toy. Since the parents won't likely lose their stars by wetting their clothes, they will take their daughter to the store to watch them claim toys while she observes. In one or two days, the four year old is likely to comply.

Another useful technique, though for older kids (ten to twelve, up through young adulthood), is Behavioral Contracting.

Behavioral Contracting – Basic Principles

Behavioral Contracting is a useful technique for older kids (usually ten to twelve years of age or older) who can be motivated to achieve a set goal. It's also a way of substituting a seductive, kid-oriented goal for an "adult" goal that a kid does NOT find intrinsically attractive. For example, many kids don't find the goal of achieving high grades in school in order to [get a higher paying job later] attractive enough to motivate them. But, achieving high grades in school to [get a dirt bike] may be immensely more appealing! Behavioral Contracting is an effective way to structure this type of goal modification so that:

- There is no confusion about the goal that has been agreed upon

  o This means the goal must be precisely defined. In the example above, the goal would be higher grades, but specifically "B-level or above" might be required.

- There is no confusion about the time frame required to reach the goal.

In the example above, "on your next report card" might be the time frame.

- There is no confusion about the reward for achieving the goal.

  o The dirt bike in the example above might be a model examined and mutually agreed upon before completing the contract.

Behavioral Contracting is much like the Positive Reinforcement Star Chart you read about earlier, except that older kids don't need the "token" stars to remind them each step of the way that they're working toward a goal. Both techniques may be "wired" in the Deflection, Diversion or Drawing modes for Word Language Commands. The Deflection mode is most effective for kids who are doing things they're not supposed to do, while the Diversion and Drawing modes are most effective for kids who aren't doing things they're supposed to do.

Behavioral Contracts need to be written out, with a copy for the parent and one for the kid to avoid arguments later. Indeed, one of the most common complaints kids direct at parents (and one to avoid if you want to retain credibility) is, "You didn't keep your promise!"

Let's examine some ways to structure Behavioral Contracts.

Behavioral Contracting for One-Time Goals

Imagine that "Devon", aged 12 years, is a seventh grade student who has always gotten "average" grades in his major subjects in school. In past years, Devon stayed home from school very infrequently and only when ill.

Three months ago, Devon's Dad was lost to a heart attack and Devon's Mom became a single parent. The many difficult adjustments imposed on the family resulted in Depression for both Mom and Devon, for which each required psychiatric care and medication. Both have made considerable progress in dealing with their loss. Devon's therapist has determined that Devon fears something will happen to his Mom at home while he's in school.

Devon has visited the School Nurse two or three times a week and is often sent home with "stomachaches." He has missed ten days of school in the past six weeks. After Devon's Pediatrician determines he is physically healthy, Mom is advised by the School Psychologist to devise a Behavioral Contract for Devon to resume regular school attendance.

With the help of the School Psychologist, Mom constructs a Behavioral Contract in the Diversion mode. You will recall that "wiring" Action Language Commands in the Diversion mode offers a kid two or more acceptable good/kidding choices to achieve rewards which together overpower the kid's anticipated "reward" for *mis*/kidding. In this instance, Devon anticipates the misdirected "reward" of staying home from school with Mom to assuage his fear of her sudden loss. By substituting an opportunity for Devon to be with Mom during the day in school, one reward can be fashioned that is both acceptable and as appealing as the misdirected goal of staying home with Mom. However, another, bigger reward can also be offered for Devon to choose NOT to spend time with Mom during the school day. Keeping in mind the overwhelming power of Superaffection as a consequence of good/kidding, Devon's reward to ignore Mom's presence in school and remain in class is a weekend trip with Mom to a special event, such as a visit to an amusement park.

Here's how such a Behavioral Contract could be constructed:

Mom arranges a schedule with the School Nurse, spanning three weeks. During the first week, Mom arranges to be in the Nurse's office at the school between 10:00 AM and Noon for the five school days; the second week for Monday, Wednesday and Friday and the third week, only on Friday. She advises Devon that arrangements have been made for him to leave class and join her there, if he feels he must, but that she will be disappointed in him if he chooses to do so. She also advises him that going to the amusement park requires him to visit the Nurse's office no more than three times the first week, no more than one time the second week and not at all the third week.

A written contract is given to Devon spanning the three weeks. He is to carry it with him in school. The contract lays out the number of "acceptable" visits to the Nurse's office each week and a pamphlet from the park is stapled to the bottom. After visiting the Nurse's office twice the first week and assuring himself Mom is really there, Devon is successfully able to remain in class the second and third weeks.

Another set of rewards for Devon's Behavioral Contract in the Diversion mode might utilize the same visitation arrangement for Mom, but substitute the reward of a video game [cassette] for incomplete compliance with the required number of days in class and the [cassette with its video player] for successful compliance.

Usually, school refusal is a *mis*/kidding issue that, once resolved, doesn't recur. However, if it were to recur, and for any form of ongoing *mis*/kidding, Behavioral Contracting can be modified to offer Rewards That "Eat." Here's how they work:

Behavioral Contracting Using Rewards That "Eat"

Imagine that several weeks after successfully remaining in class, Devon reverts to visiting the School Nurse's office several times a week. Once again, Mom constructs a Behavioral Contract, but now uses a Reward That "Eats."

Devon is advised that he may earn a cell phone if he is able to remain in class for three weeks without visiting the School Nurse during class hours. His three weeks of compliance will restart from any day he "breaks" and visits the Nurse during class hours. During those three weeks, however, he may visit the Nurse at lunchtime without penalty and speak briefly with Mom by phone from the Nurse's office.

When Devon has remained in class for three weeks without a "break", he gets a cell phone. A cell phone is a Reward That "Eats" because someone has to keep paying a monthly connection charge. Devon is advised that after he gets his cell phone he must pay 1/30th of the monthly charge (from his allowance or savings, if he has either) for any day he misses class. If he has no money, the phone is disconnected from service that month. These details are written down to avoid any misunderstandings.

Here are other Rewards That "Eat"

- Devices connected to the Internet

- Devices that require downloads

- Devices that require cassettes
- Devices that require electrical connections
- Devices with periodic service charges
- Activities that require someone to drive to a location

Another form of Behavioral Contracting could be called Constructing the Whole. Here's an example:

Behavioral Contracting To Construct the Whole

Most adults have learned early in their careers that complex and satisfying goals usually require persistent effort over time. This is not well understood by many kids, but it's easy to teach.

Imagine that Johnny, age ten years, wants his own computer. Now, he uses his older brother's machine, but only on his brother's schedule.

Johnny's bedroom looks like a garbage dump. Getting him to put toys and clothes where they belong is a constant struggle for his parents. They decide to devise a Behavioral Contract to Construct the Whole.

Johnny is given a Xeroxed card with (the same) two items listed each day. Item #1 is: Put all dirty clothes in the hamper_____. Item #2 is: Put away your toys_____. At bedtime each night Johnny must give a card to Mom or Dad with a checkmark next to each item, indicating he's completed that task. The cards are collected and counted. When Johnny has seven sequential cards completed, detailing his successful completion of these two tasks for an uninterrupted week, the contract details he gets a computer mouse. When he has fourteen sequential days, he gets a computer keyboard. Twenty-eight sequential days earns the monitor and forty-two days earns the CPU.

Since computers are Rewards That "Eat", the contract can also detail a "disconnect" consequence for failure to continue to perform these chores.

Before we close this chapter, let's take a look at a couple of forms of *Mid*/kidding that border on *KILLER*/kidding and some effective techniques to control them.

Techniques To Control Biting, Headbanging or Hairpulling

- Biting

Young kids (eighteen months to three years) who bite other kids may have In/kidding conditions that trigger anger or defensiveness (like Bipolar Disorder or Autistic Spectrum Disorders) or impulsivity (like ADHD), but the act of biting is always an inappropriate choice. This means there is always an Out/kidding component to biting and the decision to bite can be controlled by Action Language Consequences.

An effective way to control biting is to visit a toy store and purchase a cheap, unpadded (that is, *uncomfortable*) plastic football helmet with mouth visor and a tight snap-strap (difficult for a kid to remove). It's not necessary to say anything when it is snapped into place after a biting episode. The helmet "speaks" for itself in the Deterrence mode. It achieves two goals at once; it provides an uncomfortable consequence for the perpetrator and it protects potential victims. The helmet should stay in place for a sufficient time for a kid to become unhappy with its presence, like 30 minutes. Future episodes typically respond to the mere appearance of the helmet!

• Headbanging

Headbanging is usually due to an underlying In/kidding condition. The significance of headbanging can range from a variation of normal development and which will be outgrown, to a symptom of very abnormal development (as with Mental Retardation or Rett Syndrome).

Since kids do not engage in In/kidding by choice, the use of a helmet must be focused on preventing injury rather than presenting consequences. The use of a helmet for headbanging is quite effective for the limited purpose of avoiding injury to the kid. The helmet should be comfortable and well padded.

• Hairpulling

Like headbanging, hairpulling is usually a symptom of In/kidding and as such is not solely amenable to the imposition of consequences. If the scalp is the target of the hairpulling a helmet will be effective while it is worn. To the extent that hairpulling has become a habit rather than a symptom of an In/kidding condition, the habit can gradually be extinguished by using the combination of a helmet and flexible elbow splints (like plastic, toy shin splints with Velcro binders) to limit elbow flexibility and access to the hair.

Since the helmet and elbow splints are likely to be viewed by kids as "punishments" for conditions over which they have little direct control, these devices should be presented as a path to rewards in the Divergence mode using either Star Charts or Behavioral Contracts to structure their use.

For example, if twelve year old Alicia pulls her hair at night, she may be engaged in a Behavioral Contract with a Reward That Eats in the Divergence mode in which, if she agrees to wear a helmet at night for a month, she can earn a cell phone. If she elects to use the helmet with elbow restraints, her parents pay for half the monthly service fee. If she succeeds in controlling the hairpulling with regrowth of her hair, her parents pay the entire monthly service fee. As with all contracts, the details are written out to avoid confusion or misunderstanding.

As you can see, Star Charts and Behavioral Contracts are limited only by your imagination. These techniques teach kids that good/kidding efforts are rewarded, that perseverance is required for bigger rewards and that there are unpleasant consequences to *mis*/kidding. They offer opportunities for parents to engage in the HoNoR Role by responding Honestly to kidding choices, offering Nurturance in the form of love at all times while doling out (Super)affection when it is deserved and holding kids Responsible for the consequences of their acts.

Appendix III

How to Hire & When to Fire Professionals

In the Preface to this book, we introduced you to three Idiocies:

- The Permissive Idiocy: *Mis*/kidding is the expression of kids' inalienable right to do as they please. The world must adjust because kids know better than adults and controlling *mis*/kidding crushes their spirits.

- The Protective Idiocy: Kids are too frail and too dumb to learn from the consequences of *mis*/kidding. Parents who don't protect their kids from those consequences lose their love.

- The Professional Idiocy: Professionals know the TRUTH about everything. Only professionals can recognize and solve *mis*/kidding problems without crushing kids or turning off their love, so parents can't fire them or judge their competence or success in solving *mis*/kidding problems.

Up to this point in *MIS*/KIDDING we've shown how you can safely and effectively recognize, categorize and manage *mis*/kidding when you've determined it to be Out/kidding. Bypassing the first two Idiocies, you've learned to hold kids responsible for the consequences of their acts when they make significant *mis*/kidding choices, and to do so without injuring them or sacrificing their love.

You've learned when to suspect In/kidding, the *mis*/kidding that kids can't control and which usually requires the assistance of a Professional helper.

Now it's time to learn how to choose and manage those Professionals. The opinions I present in this chapter are mine and mine alone. They are based on serving at the interface of many professions, including Medicine, Psychiatry, Psychology and Education for more than forty years. My opinions do not necessarily reflect the positions of any of the "official" Professional Societies.

The advice that follows is founded on my experiences over the years as both a recipient and a provider of professional services and aims to keep *you* in control of what happens to your kid. It also aims to limit the part each Professional plays in solving *mis*/kidding problems to that professional's area of expertise and to allow you to decide when and if the *mis*/kidding issue is adequately resolved.

Let's begin with choosing and managing Physicians.

How to Hire A Physician

Physicians have completed college, where they learned the rudiments of the workings of living things, then medical school, where they learned the basics of the workings of the human body and mind. Medical school does not equip its new graduates to manage the conditions for which a parent might consult a "specialist." That knowledge is acquired by years of additional "post-graduate" study and training in specialty areas.

You've probably heard the joke, "What do they call the medical student who graduates with the lowest grade in his class?" The answer: "Doctor"! Both because of what might be called the normal "spread" of acceptable competence of medical knowledge and the isolation imposed by years of advanced learning, the possibility exists that when you consult a physician for a *mis*/kidding problem, that specialist will be unequipped to manage the problem.

Problem: "Satisfactory Competence" Is Sometimes Unacceptable In A Physician

As an example of how satisfactory competence is sometimes unacceptable in a physician, take the case of Developmental Delay. Some very proficient Psychiatrists may be unaware of one or another rare condition that results in Developmental Delay, but which causes progressive injury to the brain. One such condition, Maple Syrup Urine disease, requires definitive dietary intervention to stop its deadly progression.

Most parents will be even less familiar with Maple Syrup Urine disease than a Psychiatrist, but you can avoid the effect of unacceptable "satisfactory competence" in this case and most others by choosing your physicians beginning with "generalists", then progressing to the "specialists" till the question of In/kidding vs. Out/kidding has been answered. This means starting with your Pediatrician, moving along, if necessary, to a Neurologist and even a Geneticist to rule out physical conditions, then proceeding to a Psychiatrist for "non-physical" psychiatric conditions causing In/kidding.

Problem: Advanced Learning Can Isolate A Physician From "Real" Life

The isolation of advanced learning is created during the many years of preparation required to become a physician-"specialist." During these years a physician is often removed from the mundane worries of a typical parent, raising typical kids. Though the physician may acquire all the knowledge required to become a certified specialist, the wisdom needed to apply that knowledge and the ability to communicate that knowledge effectively and efficiently may be deficient.

For example, in one form of the Professional Idiocy, a competent physician may all but ignore your concerns when you describe your kid's problem and might proceed to suggest evaluating or treating conditions that are unrelated to the In/kidding. The end result of poor communication with your physician will be expensive, time-consuming and ultimately unsuccessful in answering the basic questions, "Does my kid have control over the *mis*/kidding (that is, is it In/kidding or Out/kidding) and if not, what condition is blocking control and how can it be treated?"

To reiterate, in choosing a physician there are two critical tests this professional must pass to earn your confidence. You must be sure the individual is competent to evaluate your kid's In/kidding and you must be certain that you and your physician can communicate effectively. A physician who passes one test, but fails the other cannot serve you well.

Judging the Competence Of A Physician

Judging the competence of a physician can seem like an insurmountable obstacle to a lay person. Actually, in this Internet Age, there are many helpful and reliable resources to accomplish this task.

Begin with two basic measures of competence – Licensing and Lawsuits. Your physician must meet certain Federal and State requirements while continuing to stay up-to-date on new medical knowledge in order to be relicensed at periodic intervals. Reports of these achievements are public knowledge. Serious (and sometimes not-so-serious) disagreements with patients and bad outcomes resulting in lawsuits are monitored and also made public. Documentation of these basic measures can most easily be found and examined on the American Medical Association website: http://www.ama-assn.org.

Judging How Well A Physician Communicates

This test begins with your first encounter. You must judge how easy or difficult it is to reach your physician, either in person with an appointment, or by phone. "Extra credit" is given for "off-hours" accessibility and weekend availability. Demerits are subtracted for being shunted off to receptionist after receptionist, answering services during standard hours or being required to rehash basic facts with a Nurse or Physician's Assistant in lieu of your physician.

You'll want to know whether your physician agrees to advise you of critical lab results in a timely fashion and whether copies of your kid's consults and lab tests will be made readily available to you as well as to other physicians working with your kid. Failure to make results available to critical parties, including you, is like not having completed the consultation at all, though you can be sure you'll be charged for the "service."

You need to be sure your physician is willing to explain in advance the strategy and anticipated steps that will be taken to answer the In/kidding vs. Out/kidding question. To glean this information from your physician, you need to ask, "How do you plan to go about finding out if my kid has a "condition" that is causing this [*mis*/kidding]? How long will it take to get answers? Will you tell me when and if you think we'll need to consult other physicians before doing so?"

Finally, "Likeability" contributes to successful communication. Speaking with others, when possible, who have consulted this physician is always helpful. As an alternative, several search engines on the Internet report patient satisfaction surveys and even "score" physicians on many above-mentioned parameters.

Remember, the fruits of competence without effective communication are expense without usable results.

After you've consulted with one or more physicians to either discover or rule out physical illnesses and conditions that take away kids' choice-making, you may need to proceed to a Psychologist for additional Professional assistance. Just as you did with the physicians you consulted, you'll want to choose and manage psychologists to get the help you want while staying in control of the process.

Choosing & Managing Psychologists

Psychologists are often asked to identify or define mental illnesses that are not under kids' control and which take away kids' choice-making; in other words, mental conditions that cause In/kidding. Such conditions include psychiatric illnesses, Developmental Delay and Mental Retardation, Learning Disabilities and Autistic Spectrum Disorders.

In this sense, psychologists share responsibility with physicians in recognizing many forms of In/kidding. Unlike physicians, however, psychologists are not asked to diagnose or treat physical illnesses that present as In/kidding. Since In/kidding always raises the possibility of physical illness, whenever you suspect In/kidding, you must consult a physician to rule out physical conditions *before* consulting a psychologist.

Two other facets of the psychologist's training are measuring kids' capabilities and the degree to which kids' achievements fall short of their capabilities. Delineating any discrepancy between a kid's achievement and a kid's ability defines the goals of that kid's educational strategies and provides the means for determining the success or failure of those strategies. Without these measures, Educators will squander their resources and encounter frustration in trying to reach ill-defined social and academic goals for your kid.

Finally, though you've already learned how to "wire" Word language Commands in Chapter Four and how to energize them with Action Language Consequences in Chapter Five, psychologists can provide professional assistance in managing *mis*/kidding and developing kids' motivation and insight through counseling and therapy.

How to Choose the Right Psychologist

As you've seen above, Psychologists can diagnose mental conditions not under kids' control. They can measure kids' capabilities and delineate discrepancies between kids' abilities and their level of achievement. They can interpret their findings to parents and Educators, helping parents to better understand their kids' individual needs and helping educators to develop plans and strategies to meet kids' special needs. Finally, psychologists can counsel kids and parents who need help coping with physical, mental or educational challenges.

Although all psychologists are familiar with the techniques required to perform the services mentioned above, some "species" of psychologists are more proficient than others at achieving one or another of these duties. For example, psychologists who have reached the "Doctoral" level (i.e. Ph.D.'s) may be expected to have a wider experience in all the areas of service listed, while Masters level psychologists (i.e. M.A.) likely have greater capabilities than Bachelor level psychologists (i.e. B.A. or B.S.), but less than PhD's.

Bachelor level psychologists, often called Psychometrists (i.e. "Mind-measurers") can reliably administer tests of Intellectual Ability (i.e. I.Q. tests), Achievement and Social Maturity, but usually do not have the required training and experience to diagnose mental illness or provide psychotherapy. Psychometrists are often employed by schools to perform tests for the purpose of developing Individualized Educational Plans (i.e. IEP's) and other educational strategies. Because Psychometrists "wear two hats" (advocate for both the school and your kid), their recommendations may be influenced more by what services the school has available than strictly by what your kid needs.

Doctoral psychologists are more professionally independent than Masters level psychologists or Bachelor level psychologists. This means they can more easily act as your kid's advocate, especially if your kid requires services not readily available through the school. These highly trained psychologists can measure, interpret and counsel at any level required by their findings.

My recommendations for choosing a psychologist are listed below:

Recommended "Species" Of Psychologists For Various Services

Level of Training	Administering Tests	Advising Teams of Educators	Counseling & Therapy	Diagnosing Mental Illness
Ph.D.	+	+	+	+
Masters	+	+	+/-	+/-
Bachelor	+	+/-	+/-	-

The Difference between "School Psychologists" and "Private Psychologists"

In addition to the different "species" of psychologists outlined above, psychologists may be found in various "habitats." As I've mentioned, lesser trained psychologists are likely to be less independent from their employer (such as a school) than more highly trained psychologists. You are more likely to ensure advocacy for your kid the more highly trained the psychologist you consult. Even so, School Psychologists even at the Doctorate level are, by definition, employees of schools and are obligated by their employer to consider the resources and budget of the school when proposing appropriate services for your kid. This means their recommendations are likely to be flavored to at least some extent by the school's staffing or budgetary limitations. The result may be a proposal for a less costly service or one for which the school has staffing rather than a more appropriate, though more costly or more staff-intensive service. This conundrum can be avoided by consulting a psychologist in private practice.

Though Private Psychologists are not "free" like School Psychologists, their allegiance is directed entirely at you and your kid. If you have doubts about your kid's abilities, special needs or performance levels as they are presented to you by your kid's school or are contesting a strategy the school has proposed, you are best advised to employ a Private, Ph.D.-level Clinical Child Psychologist. Only this "species" of independent, highly trained professional, removed from the "habitat" of the school can advocate for your kid and assist you in formulating the best educational strategy for your kid.

Choosing & Managing Educators

Educators are arguably the most diverse group of professionals and their capabilities are certainly the most wide-ranging. Each link in the chain of learning skills your kid needs to master on the journey to adulthood has generated its own educational specialist. Here follows a list of some of those specialized Educators:

- Teachers for each grade level
- Perceptual Motor Specialists
- Special Education teachers
- Speech & Language Clinicians
- Reading Specialists
- School Psychologists
- Audiologists
- Physical Education teachers
- Pupil Personnel Workers
- Principals

It's no surprise that a "team" of specialized Educators gathered, for example, to generate an Individualized Educational Plan (I.E.P.) in your school for your kid, might intimidate you and make you feel you have no control over the process of providing for your kid's educational needs. But these professionals, like the Physicians and Psychologists we've discussed previously, are your employees and may be "hired" or "fired", depending upon your determination of their competence and effectiveness in solving your kid's educational problem. True, Educators, like Physicians and Psychologists, have special knowledge they can bring to bear in diagnosing and managing educational needs. But you as a parent have special knowledge of your kid and have rejected the Professional Idiocy. Using the *Mis*/kidding

Process, you are quite capable of deciding if a group of Educators are getting the job done and, if not, how and when you will replace them.

In the paragraphs that follow, let's re-examine some principles you've met earlier in *MIS*/KIDDING and apply them in this context.

Begin With The Question, "Is there ANY educational problem?"

An educational problem is merely another form of *mis*/kidding. That being the case, the question really translates to, "Is my kid *mis*/kidding?" As you learned in Chapter One, *mis*/kidding is identified by consulting the Consequence Areas – Age Work, Others, Authority. If your kid is working at grade level (that is, at the grade level for your kid's age), the test of Age Work has been passed. If Others are not, for the most part, complaining about your kid and your kid, for the most part, enjoys being with classmates, the test of Others has been passed. Finally, if your kid follows most reasonable school rules, the test of Authority has been passed. Any kid who passes all three "tests" is NOT *mis*/kidding, has NO educational problem and requires NO intervention by you, by Educators or by anyone else. You need only follow the *Mis*/kidding Process to make this determination and no professional assistance is necessary.

Follow By Asking, "If there's mis/kidding in school, how severe is it?"

This is where you determine the level of the *mis*/kidding, as you've learned to do in Chapter Two. You'll count up the number of Consequence Areas affected by the *mis*/kidding to decide how much time you have to intervene. For example, dangerous bullying, either by or of your kid, which may have reached the level of *KILLER*/kidding, needs to be STOPPED IMMEDIATELY, without waiting to find out causes. Conversely, *mis*/kidding at the *mini*/kidding level, such as an occasional nasty comment to or from your kid, may be ignored. Finally, *mis*/kidding at the *Mid*/kidding level, such as failing several subjects or refusing to attend school, will require management achieved in a stepwise fashion over time.

Now, Find Out If The Mid/kidding In School Is In/kidding Or Out/kidding

Following the principles you've acquired in Chapter Three, decide if your kid might be In/kidding; that is, engaging in *mis*/kidding that your kid cannot control. If you suspect In/kidding, you must find out whether you need to adjust to your kid's innate limitations or whether your kid has a "condition", such as Asperger Disorder, ADHD or Dyslexia, requiring professional diagnosis and treatment. Remember, when In/kidding is a possibility, you will want to follow the professional path of Physician > Psychologist > Educator. Skipping over the Physician or the Psychologist and turning first to Educators, runs the risk of missing a condition Educators cannot identify or manage, such as a Seizure Disorder, Bipolar Disorder or Autism.

If you suspect Out/kidding, remember that this form of *mis*/kidding can be controlled by your kid and that it represents bad choice-making by your kid. Even when Out/kidding occurs in school, you can manage it by "wiring" good/kidding commands as you learned in Chapter Four and "energizing" them with Action Language Consequences as you learned in Chapter Five.

What To Do If You Disagree With The School's Strategy, Or It's Not Working

Here's a list of reasons you might consider firing your kids' Educators:

- You disagree with the Educators' strategy for managing the *mis*/kidding.

  o It's the wrong teacher

  o It's the wrong class

  o It's the wrong school

  o The school is too far away

  o The school isn't safe

- You disagree with the Educators' assessment of your kid's capabilities.

- You disagree with the Educators' assessment of your kid's special needs.

- No progress or too slow progress has occurred over a reasonable period of time.

Each one of these determinations is *yours* to make. To be sure your conclusion is accurate; you'll need to have reliable answers to each of these basic questions:

1. Does my kid have a "condition" that limits good/kidding?

2. Does the school need to accommodate any such condition?

3. What is my kid's educational capability; that is, what's the best my kid can do?

4. How does what my kid is doing educationally compare to the best my kid can do; specifically, how many grade levels apart are my kid's ability level and my kid's achievement level?

5. If there's a difference between ability level and achievement level, how long should it reasonably take for my kid to catch up (or for the *mis*/kidding to resolve)?

What To Do If You're Missing An Answer To One Of The Above 5 "Basic Questions"?

Without well-documented (written) answers to each of the five "basic questions", generated by one or more of the Physician(s) and/or Psychologists you consulted before you turned to the Educators, you will not, as a lay person, be able to effectively redirect the educational strategy. If you're missing an answer, you'll need to go back to a Physician or Psychologist to get it. This is critical because you will need a Physician or a Psychologist's knowledge to challenge professional Educators. Once you've acquired this documentation, only two outcomes are possible:

 • The Educators will incorporate the new information into a new educational strategy and provide you with an answer to question #5.

OR

 • The Educators will NOT incorporate the new information into a new educational strategy and will leave you guessing the answer to question #5.

When a new educational strategy is devised, you must hold the Educators to the answer they gave you to question #5; that is, how long should it reasonably take for my kid to catch up or for the *mis*/kidding to resolve?

When Educators cannot or will not accommodate to your kid's needs or refuse to incorporate critical professional recommendations into a new educational strategy, *it's time to fire them.*

How & Why to "Fire" Your Kid's Educators

Sometimes you will encounter a teacher who can't relate to your kid or a class that is unsuitable for your kid's special needs. Sometimes your kid's classmates will make the class an inappropriate milieu for comfortable learning. Occasionally, a school will not have the resources or commitment to provide the services your Physician or Psychologist consultants have deemed necessary for your kid.

In any of these cases, if you've made reasonable efforts to enlist the help of the Educators and are not met with success, it may be time to fire those Educators or even withdraw from the school. This is not as difficult as it might seem and your determination to extract the full benefits of schooling from your kid's educational experience can literally be lifesaving for your kid. Remember that your kid's self-esteem is anchored to achievement and that for kids, school is the arena in which a great amount of ongoing achievement accumulates. Remember, too, that lack of self-esteem robs a kid of motivation and inevitably leads to either depression and self-injurious acts or to anger and outward-directed violence.

How to Fire a Teacher or a Class

Switching teachers or classes can potentially alienate Educators in the school, position your kid as a target of bullying by former classmates or result in your kid's placement in an even less appropriate class. Sometimes, attempting to switch teachers or classes can result in your being placed in an adversarial relationship with the teacher or other Educators. To avoid these pitfalls, you need to be sure you're making a good decision and you need to document the reasons for your decision in case you are challenged. Here are some suggestions to help you achieve your goals:

- If your Physician or Psychologist consultants have recommended services that the teacher or the class seems unable or unwilling to accommodate, be sure you fully understand those recommendations. Go back to the consultants, if necessary, and be sure their recommendations are truly CRITCAL NEEDS.

- If you are unhappy with the teacher's management of the class or the provision of services, arrange to observe your kid in class with the teacher. Be sure to write down your observations in case you are challenged. If at all possible, make the observation(s) without your kid's knowledge of your presence to avoid provoking *mis*/kidding.

- If you are considering changing teachers or classes because critical needs are not being met or the teacher is unwilling or unable to provide them, it's reasonable to meet with the teacher to discuss your observations and allow the teacher to offer solutions to your concerns. This is the time to review with the teacher any disparity between the critical needs your consultants identified and the services you've observed being rendered. This is also the time to judge whether your concerns are being taken seriously.

- If, after determining critical needs, observing the delivery of services in the classroom and offering the teacher an opportunity to redirect the services, you are convinced a change of teachers or class is necessary, you will want to determine what alternative teacher or class is available, if any. It makes no sense to move your kid randomly to another teacher or class without being sure the new teacher or class is a better fit.

• Once you've made your decision to switch and found a suitable alternative, you'll need to communicate that decision to the teacher and the principal, both in person and in writing.

Meeting these Educators face to face conveys your personal involvement in the decision.

Communicating your decision in writing gives you an opportunity to document your kid's needs, your personal classroom observations and the teacher's inadequate response to your concerns. Send a copy of your summary and conclusions to the teacher and the principal and keep a copy of your own. Try to be kind to the Educators with your summary, even if the process has generated tensions; you will likely have to work with these folks in the future.

• Once you've made arrangements to switch your kid's teacher or class, let your kid know what you have decided to do and why. This relieves your kid of any false sense of responsibility for the switch. This is important because kids, especially young kids, assume personal responsibility for most things that happen around them.

If You Must "Fire" A School

When switching teachers or classes won't or can't provide for critical educational needs for your kid, you may have to consider "firing" the school. This means switching either your kid's school or your kid's schooling program.

It is your right and responsibility to arrange for the most appropriate educational setting for your kid, even when a public school is unwilling or unable to do so. In most states, however, you do not have the option of removing a kid younger than 16 years of age from all forms of education. Doing so would meet the criteria for child neglect and would prompt authorities to intervene. Also, in some states, certain forms of alternative education are considered "neglectful." Since this varies from state to state it is critical for you to research any alternative educational plans for your kid before taking definitive action.

Here follow some options you have if you must fire your kid's school:

• Boundary Exceptions for medical, psychological or educational reasons.

• Magnet Schools & Charter Schools

- School Voucher Program
- Private, Religious & Military Schools
- Home/Hospital Programs
- Scholarship Funding Organizations
- Virtual Schooling
- Home Schooling

Boundary Exceptions for Critical Needs

If your kid has a medical, psychological or educational need that cannot be met at the current school, one option that may be available is a boundary change. All this means is that the school acknowledges that your kid's special need cannot be accommodated at your home school and, in spite of the location of your residence, your kid will be reassigned to another school as if you lived in that school's district.

To effect a boundary change, you must have adequate professional documentation of your kid's special need and the critical nature of the services unavailable at the "home" school. Even with such evidence, it may be difficult to switch schools. School administrators have to consider budgetary restraints, transportation factors and overcrowding, among other things, at the recipient school and these considerations may negate the possibility of a switch.

Charter & Magnet Schools

Charter Schools are public schools that have greater freedom to determine their curriculum, educational goals and means of achieving them than traditional public schools. The term "charter" derives from the contract under which these schools must operate and which removes the schools from the usual school administrative pathways.

Charter schools must hire accredited teachers and staff, abide by state health and safety regulations and meet their state's graduation requirements just as any public school. Like any other schools, charter schools vary widely in student outcomes. Most charter schools publicize their successes, often on the internet, thus allowing you as a parent to research the pros and cons of enrolling your kid. The more successful charter schools boast many applicants for each available seat. Gaining entrance to many charter schools can be difficult.

To find a charter school for your kid, begin by asking your kid's home school for information. Your district's school administrators may be helpful as well. Finally, charter school directories for your area are usually available on the Net along with contact information, school grades and other specific details. One especially helpful website devoted to charter schools is: www.uscharterschools.org.

Magnet Schools are public schools that are often outside your kid's "home school" zone. Unlike charter schools, magnet schools remain within the public school administrative pathway and do not operate independently. Historically, the term "magnet" applied to the goal of such schools to "attract" students of all races and backgrounds and so voluntarily create diversity.

These days, magnet schools, like charter schools, have become competitive for students with areas of talent corresponding to the school's focused curriculum. Some special areas of focus include math, science and the arts. Since enrollment in magnet schools is competitive, higher achieving students are more likely to gain entrance. Indeed, in most locales, only a percentage of applicants gain admittance.

To learn more about magnet schools within your kid's area, begin by asking your kid's home school for information. As with charter schools, your district's school administrators may be helpful in getting you started. One internet site that is especially helpful in learning about charter schools is: http://www.magnet.edu.

School Voucher Programs

School vouchers are payments made to you as a parent, either by your state or, sometimes, the federal government to fund part of the cost of a private school for your kid. Once received, the money may be used for any accredited school, even a religious school.

Vouchers have aroused intense debate wherever they have been proposed. Some feel they threaten public schools, either by reducing their funding or by drawing away their best students. Others feel their kids can "fire" a bad school and pay, at least in part, for a better one.

There is no uniformity in voucher programs from one locale to another. Only diligent research into voucher options in your area will determine their availability. As with the options mentioned above, your kid's school administrators and local government officials will be able to get you started finding critical answers.

Private, Religious & Military Schools

Private schools are independently administered schools which establish their own criteria for admission and are financed to some degree by tuition charged to their students. Many such schools offer scholarships to needy students to ease tuition costs. Private schools generally conform to state and local public school regulations, though the degree to which they conform is worth researching carefully before enrolling your kid.

One subcategory of private schools is religious schools, which like other public schools; generally conform to state and local public school regulations.

Religious schools add to the basic studies a religious curriculum which is unavailable in public schools.

Another subcategory of private schools is military schools, which like religious schools, generally provide a curriculum conforming to state and local regulations, but superimpose a form of military-style discipline. Military school can be lifesaving for some types of *mis*/kidding.

One very useful website you can review for more details on private schools and which may help you find a school with a good "fit" for your kid is: www.privateschoolreview.com.

Home/Hospital (H/H) Programs

H/H programs are designed to continue education for students who are usually temporarily unable to attend public school due to a physical or mental health issue. There are strict requirements for H/H status determined by state or local government. These include limits on the duration of services. In some cases, the total allotted time for a student's duration of services may be used either as a block of time or may be used intermittently up to the designated total.

H/H status requires professional (usually a physician) documentation of diagnosis and anticipated length of absence. An Individualized Educational Program (IEP) team at the home school may need to meet and authorize H/H status.

While temporary removal from the public classroom may enable a student to recover from physical illness or enable mental health issues to receive intense treatment, long-term removal of a student from interaction with peers in class can result in isolation and ostracism.

Applying for H/H begins with a professional consultation to establish a diagnosis and a rationale for the program as well as an estimate of length of absence. The school is then consulted for approval and arrangements.

Scholarship Funding Organizations(SFO's)

Scholarship Funding Organizations (SFO's) are non-profit organizations that issue scholarships and determine student eligibility for tuition assistance. Many states support SFO's through tax write-offs and many wealthy people contribute to SFO's either during life or through their estates, not only for the benefit of needy students, but also in support of students with specific attributes. For example, scholarship funds may be available for children of soldiers killed in Afghanistan or Iraq. Some funds may be designated for use only at a specific school, while others may be cash scholarships for use at any school.

Since there are so many SFO's, repeated web searches are advisable to uncover possibilities for your kid.

Virtual Schooling

Virtual or Cyberschools are generally full-time, accredited schools operating either under the aegis of the local public school system or owned and funded privately. These schools span all grades and must abide by tight standards and regulations.

Internet technology allows for interaction between student and teacher from afar, whether at home or in another part of a physical school. Usually, but not always, the required software to run the program and instructional basic materials are provided by state or local funding. Occasionally, students must pay fees for these materials.

Virtual schooling may be fulltime at home or split between home and the public school. It can be an attractive option for kids who are physically or emotionally threatened by attending their home school or whose emotional instability may pose a threat to others.

As with H/H programs, in which students are separated from physical interaction with peers, isolation is a potential downside. For kids lacking in social skills, full-time virtual schooling may exacerbate social deficits.

Home Schooling (H/S)

Home schooling is the most definitive option you have to "fire" your kid's school. H/S offers an almost infinite variety of learning styles you can "fit" to your kid. The price you pay is twofold: It can be expensive and it will be time-consuming. Indeed, since at least one parent's time must be heavily committed to teaching, the potential time remaining to that parent for other critical activities, including employment, will be curtailed.

H/S can better prepare your kid for college, strengthen family bonds and individualize your kid's education to fit specific goals and talents. Because H/S is heavily regulated to ensure a minimum equivalency to public education, you must satisfy your local government that the H/S curriculum will be adequate and that you are able to administer it. The preparation and requirements for H/S in each state varies widely, but one excellent website devoted to helping you organize and carry out H/S may be found at: www.homeschool.com.

About the Author

Dr. Alan Davick, a Developmental-Behavioral Pediatrician, has taught parents and professional colleagues how to recognize and manage complex misbehavior in children for 40 years.

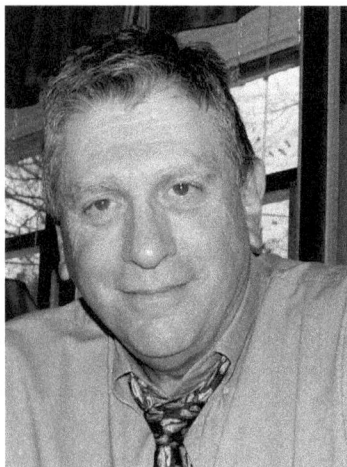

Trained at the Johns Hopkins Medical Institutions, Dr. Davick has maintained clinical practice throughout those years. He has, as a Major in the Army Medical Corps, served as Pediatrician-in-Chief at Tuttle Army Health Clinic, Savannah GA and later, while engaged in private Pediatric practice, as Behavioral-Developmental Consultant to the Chatsworth School for Exceptional Children, in Baltimore County, MD.

Dr. Davick has focused his knowledge and experience on separating innate conditions like ADHD, Bipolar Disorder, Cerebral Palsy, Developmental Delay and Epilepsy, masquerading as willful misbehavior, from truly volitional misconduct, like Oppositional-Defiant Disorder and Conduct Disorders.

Ordering Information

For more information about Dr. Davick's books, please send your queries to:

Alan M. Davick, M.D.
MISKIDDING, LLC
P.O. Box 101127
Cape Coral, FL 33910-1127

URL: www.miskidding.com
Email: miskidding1@gmail.com

Alan M. Davick

Alan M. Davick

Alan M. Davick

www.ingramcontent.com/pod-product-compliance
Lightning Source LLC
Chambersburg PA
CBHW080608270326
41928CB00016B/2967